PRAISE FOR

M000106624

"*Disconnect* raises significant questions about our constant exposure to the electronic radiation that flows from the devices into our homes, workplace, and public spaces."

— *The Washington Post*

"*Disconnect.* . . is just as courageous and groundbreaking as Rachel Carson's *Silent Spring*. It could save even more lives."

— Tracy Fernandez Rysavy, Green America

"Devra Davis presents a range of recent and long-suppressed research in this timely bombshell. Cell phone radiation is a national emergency. Stunningly, the most popular gadget of our age has now been shown to damage DNA, break down the brain's defenses, and reduce sperm count while increasing memory loss, the risk of Alzheimer's disease, and even cancer. The growing brains of children make them especially vulnerable."

— Barnes & Noble

"The story behind the story needs to be told. . . . For the sake of our children and grandchildren, we should promote simple precautions to reduce direct exposure to the brain by using headsets, speaker phones, and texting. This will protect us from whatever health hazards may emerge decades later and also encourage safer development of this revolutionary technology in the meantime."

— *The Huffington Post*

"This book should be required reading, particularly for parents. It will make you uncomfortable. But it may spur you to immediately change your cell phone habits and those of your children."

— Diane Makovsky, *The Free Lance-Star*

"From tobacco smoke to chemical pollutants to climate change, Dr. Devra Davis has been in the vanguard of the environmental health frontier. Her experience shedding light on man-made preventable environmental hazards makes the 2023 expanded edition of *Disconnect* all the more compelling since her original warnings on the biological and environmental effects of cellular radiation are finally raising the alarms that they warrant."

— Mikhail Kogan, MD, Medical Director, George Washington University Center for Integrative Medicine, Associate Professor of Medicine, George Washington University, and founder and member of the Board, AIM Health Institute.

"Cellular radiation and the onslaught of 5G is more problematic than most people realize. As Devra Davis keenly explains in *Disconnect*, it is urgent that parents, school leaders, elected officials, philanthropists and even our environmental health warriors find the bandwidth to lean into this topic and demand safer alternatives to wireless and the thousands of mini cell towers now permeating our landscapes."

— Lendri Purcell, Vice President of Jonas Philanthropies.

"*Disconnect* is an important book both for the general public and for scientists, researchers, policymakers, and politicians. Anyone who cares about public health must read."

— Linda S. Birnbaum, PhD, DABT, Scientist Emeritus and Former Director of NIEHS and NTP; Scholar in Residence at the Nicholas School of the Environment of Duke University

"If you or your loved ones have wireless devices, then you should read *Disconnect*. With her background as a uniquely accomplished scientist and public health advocate who has worked both inside and outside of government, Devra Davis offers invaluable insights on how we are now surrounded by levels of electromagnetic exposures that a strong body of science demonstrates are highly risky to public health, especially to the youngest of us. Davis explains strategies that have allowed telecom and tech industries to enjoy extraordinary growth at great risks to humanity. While the narrative described in *Disconnect* might seem unbelievable to some, it is recognizable to those familiar with strategies that the tobacco industry used to effectively grow or protect profits as evidence strengthened that smoking cigarettes poses serious health risks. To help our children and grandchildren inherit the best society possible, please read *Disconnect* and talk about it with others. *Disconnect* shows us the path forward."

— Sophia Ruan Gushée, author of *A to Z of D-Toxing:*
The Ultimate Guide to Reducing Our Toxic Exposures, host
of Practical Nontoxic Living podcast, and founder of Ruan
Living, a nontoxic lifestyle ecosystem.

Devra Davis is "recognized for her research on the dangers of environmental pollution, her advocacy for environmental health policies, and her work to educate the public about the importance of protecting the environment."

— Green America Lifetime Achievement Award, 2011

"By cogently detailing the profound disconnect between professional standards for measuring, monitoring and protecting wireless equipment from harmful interference, in contrast to doing the same to meet standards for exposure to humans and the environment, this critically important book provides a Northstar to guide us towards very real solutions to this ongoing dilemma."

— Joseph Sandri, JD, IEEE, President,
National Spectrum Management Association, and former
Co-President of FiberTower Corporation.

"Through bipartisan legislation, the state of New Hampshire formed a commission of independent experts tasked with finding the truth about the effects of wireless radiation. The commission findings align closely with those of *Disconnect*, delivering a message we all need to heed."

— Kent Chamberlin, PhD, Professor and Chairman Emeritus
of Electrical and Computer Engineering,
University of New Hampshire

Disconnect

A Scientist's Solutions for Safer Technology

New Expanded Edition

DEVRA DAVIS PHD MPH

Disconnect

A Scientist's Solutions for Safer Technology

Devra Davis, PhD MPH
Published by New Voices Press
75 West End Avenue Suite C19H
New York, NY 10023
307-543-1461
212-580-8833

For information contact info@ehtrust.org
phone: 307-213-9839

Library of Congress Cataloguing-in-Publication Data

Disconnect

A Scientist's Solutions for Safer Technology
Devra Davis, PhD MPH
Published by New Voices Press

978-0-9883591-8-5

1. microwave radiation 2. pediatric environmental health
3. male reproductive health 4. environmental cancer

Book cover and interior design by Tony Iatridis, nycartdirector.com

DEDICATION (2010)

*Ellie and Alan, Mindy and Dan, Ken, Les,
Lloyd, Michael and Gloria, Keith and Pam,
and their families,*

DEDICATION (2024)

Davis, Josephine Jean, Raleigh, Noa Jane, and Ruby

Contents

FOREWORD (2010)

By David Servan-Schreiber, MD, PhD (1961-2011)

If that were true, we'd know about it!

I once had a short conversation about health effects of cell phone radiation with the current and a past director of the National Cancer Institute at a cocktail party following a public talk. They both dismissed the topic offhand: "First, there's never been any evidence that electromagnetic fields can affect DNA. Thus, they simply cannot contribute to cancer risk; second epidemiological studies have never documented an increased risk of brain tumors from cell phone use; and third, there has been no increase in the global number of brain tumors, which, surely, we'd have seen given the large number of people using cell phones today." Case closed. As this book will show you, just scratching the surface of what is known about health risks of cell phone electromagnetic radiation is enough to easily dismiss all three of these arguments. I knew that at the time. So what struck me was the degree to which these two brilliant men, outstanding doctors and world-class scientists, were utterly convinced that this was not a worthwhile area of scientific inquiry. The question in my mind continues to resonate to this day: How can this be?

The best answer I've been able to come up with since then is that for most reasonable people, including the scientific leaders of our prestigious medical institutions, it is inconceivable that if cell phones caused health problems we wouldn't already know about it. "If it were true that these devices cause harm, we would know!"

I myself, a physician, a scientist, a patient being followed for a malignant brain tumor for the past eighteen years, lived with exactly the same

1

assumption. I used a cell phone just like everybody else. I had heard, like my NCI colleagues, of all the studies that had never found a convincing link between cell phone use and cancer risk. That seemed reassuring enough. I was convinced, as well, that such technology could not possibly be released on the enormous scale that it has reached today without governments having demanded proof that there could be no health hazards from the widespread use of a new type of microwave radiation that practically everyone would be intensely exposed to for decades.

In fact, I had been using my cell phone for many years, in spite of being a brain tumor patient in remission, without any self-consciousness, until an impromptu dinner with the author of this book one summer evening in Pittsburgh. Dr. Davis had recently accepted the offer to head a Center for Environmental Oncology at the university's Hillman Cancer Center and somebody had suggested we should meet. I was intrigued by the intelligence and the charm of this veteran of many courageous scientific explorations into the link between industrial practices and disastrous public health consequences. Then, my cell phone, which at that time I was carrying in my pocket, rang loudly and I noticed the horrified expression of my dinner mate when I answered the call by putting the phone directly to my ear. She practically stood up from her seat and shouted: "What? You of all people are not using an earpiece?"

After I finished my call, and gave her a quizzical look about her behavior, she asked me two plain questions that have remained engraved in my memory as the perfect conversation starter with anyone who thinks, like I did, that they "know" there cannot be a health problem with cell phone radiation:

- Did you know that most cell phones come with a notice that says "do not hold closer than one inch from your body"?
- Did you know that insurance companies refuse to provide coverage to cell phone companies and operators in case of claims of health damage from long-term operation of their devices?

2

This is when I realized how little I really knew about the "studies" so often referred to in order to dismiss any type of health concern about cell phones. And how much I was going to have to learn. I didn't stop at what Dr. Davis told me that evening. I've learned that in Science, the opinion of a single person, however smart and diligent, does not truth make. I did look up the studies. I read the thoroughly documented report of the Bioinitiative Working Group that was published in August 2007 by many of the leading scientists in this field after reviewing practically all the literature available at the time. What I found is precisely what this book describes: an immense "disconnect" between the common public and medical opinion about cell phone safety and what the data actually said.

A year later, Dr. Davis and I helped organize a consensus statement of twenty international scientists and oncologists to emphasize the importance of protecting children from cell phone exposure and the urgent need for more research on how electromagnetic fields from cell phones affect biological mechanisms sustaining health or causing disease.

I am proud today that she asked me to write the foreword for her book summarizing all she has found over the years. The politics of science and the pressures of business have not been kind to scientists such as Dr. Davis who have been among the first to call attention to a possible public health effect of new technology. We don't want to believe that our new toys to which we are so attached — and which bring in enormous profits — could also cause our demise or that of our children. But science is not about belief. Governments' responsibility to their citizens should not be either. This debate brought forth with talent, clarity, and power of argument in this book by Dr. Davis should be about facts and about our choices in view of those facts. Let us hope that this is just the kind of conversation that will be starting.

— David Servan-Schreiber, MD, PhD

Clinical Professor of Psychiatry, University of Pittsburgh; Adjunct

Professor of General Oncology, M.D. Anderson Cancer Center, University of Texas; Lecturer, School of Medicine of Lyon, France; and author of *Anticancer: A New Way of Life*

FOREWORD (2024)

By Frank Clegg

E very living thing from the simplest plants and animals to the more than eight billion humans depends on electromagnetic fields (EMF) for their existence. Each of the atoms in our bodies is attracted or repelled by the pull of these fields. Without the very low levels of natural EMF that keep our hearts beating and our minds thinking, we cannot live. So it is sheer hubris to claim that the phenomenal increase in everyday exposure levels of radio frequency EMF radiation (RF) — now greater than ever before in human history — arising from the unprecedented growth of cellular and other wireless communications has no effect on our well-being.

When I served as president of Microsoft Canada, I witnessed the incredible benefits that technological advancements can provide and the capacity of my engineering colleagues to solve previously unsolvable problems. In the past decades, my family and I also witnessed firsthand the tremendous harms that can be caused when technology is implemented without diligent consideration of its impact on human health or the environment.

The massive expansions of wireless radiation today will affect the quality of our children's and grandchildren's lives as well as the survival capacity of our natural surroundings. My concern for them and my training in engineering are the reasons why I co-founded Canadians for Safe Technology (C4ST) in 2012 after a 40+-year career spent entirely in the technology industry. It is also why I feel especially proud to provide you with this introduction to the updated 2023 edition of *Disconnect*.

Before founding C4ST, I invested a significant amount of time researching and talking with experts on this topic. They included medical and scientific researchers from Harvard, Yale, Columbia, McGill, and Trent universities, and the University of Toronto. Among these experts, Devra Davis stood out as an extremely knowledgeable and strategic thinker, with the exceptional ability to render complex scientific topics understandable.

Dr. Davis, who was a member of the team awarded the Nobel Peace Prize in 2007 with Al Gore and an award-winning scientist for her work in environmental health, was one of the very first experts I reached out to in my quest to understand the effects of RF radiation from wireless devices. Since then, she and I and many others working in the field have held a number of conferences, including presentations to Canadian and American officials and policymakers.

When *Disconnect* was first published in 2010, some leaders of the scientific community were already expressing concern about the potential impact of RF radiation on humans. Today, a growing chorus of world-renowned physicists, engineers, physicians, and other scientists has published thousands of peer-reviewed papers, including more than 270 expert scientists from 55 nations who are urging the United Nations and World Health Organization to classify wireless radio frequency radiation, including 5G, as carcinogenic to humans.

Dr. Davis, her colleagues, and I are now joined by hundreds of other experts in the field calling for international agencies to revise outdated safety standards to take into account modern-day usage of cellular equipment, especially by children. While we await those regulatory changes, in my opinion it would be irresponsible to continue delaying mitigation of critical real-world concerns. The alleged energy savings of this technology has been exposed as a carefully crafted illusion. Think about this: if the "cloud" that aims to connect 50 billion wireless devices by the end of this decade were a country, each year it would consume as much electricity as Russia. As systems become more efficient, this spurs the demand for more consumption so that gains in efficiency tend to easily be overrun by accelerated demand. While this may be a great business model, it augurs poorly for our health and that of the planet.

In 2021 I challenged a president of Rogers Communications to provide evidence to support his grossly misleading claim that the radiation from doubling antennas for 5G planned for Eastern Ontario is "very, very safe." Further, citing thousands of scientific studies showing evidence of harm, I proposed that until and unless proof of safety had been provided that his company should return the $150 million in annual government assistance received to underwrite the installation of these radiating devices. I noted that wired fiber optic cable is safer, faster, and more secure, as well as more cost-effective.

I continue to await a response to this challenge.

I am sure you have, or will have, some questions of your own. Here are queries that have not been answered by the U.S. Federal Communications Commission, nor by Health Canada or Industry Canada.

1. Why do China, India, and Russia provide protection that is up to 100 times lower maximum exposures for their citizens than those set in the United States, Canada, England, Australia, New Zealand, and some European countries?

2. Why are cell phones that exceed current outdated, low-level government regulations and guidelines on the market today in the U.S. and Canada, although some of the same phones have been recalled in France?

3. Why are the technology and telecommunication industries able to ship wireless products into the market without any safety testing or proof they are not harmful? They simply state

"this product meets government regulations if used correctly." Why are they not held to the same standards, monitoring and regular safety testing as the automotive, pharmaceutical, and chemical industries?

4. Why are our government agencies not investing more aggressively in fiber solutions? Over the long-term, fiber is significantly less capital intensive. Fiber is up to 100 times faster, more reliable and resilient, more protective of our security and privacy, has hundreds of thousands fewer points of vulnerability, and is significantly greener and more protective of our environment.

5. Why is there no analysis of the full economic burden of wireless technology: health costs, lost productivity costs, cost of security breaches, ransomware, and property damage from reduced weather forecasting ability? Why are these costs not allocated to the industries that are harvesting billions of dollars of profit and revenue growth from their devices but instead passed onto the taxpayers?

6. Why are our government agencies neither educating the public, especially parents and teachers, about the potential harmful effects from wireless devices and their supporting infrastructure nor advising us how to use devices more safely?

7. Why are the governments of Canada and the U.S. relying on last century approaches that override local control and rapidly approving and siting more than a million new antennas for 5G being erected in the U.S. and Canada, some of which are more than three stories tall and posted within a few feet of bedrooms and schoolrooms?

It has been more than a decade since I joined Dr. Davis's team at Environmental Health Trust (EHT) as co-chair of the Business Advisory Group. I now sit on the board of directors. I am grateful to her, EHT's indomitable executive director. Theodora Scarato, and their many colleagues for their incredible work. Environmental Health Trust is one of the best resources in the world for information regarding the effects of RF radiation, key published research, and updates on judicial decisions, community actions, and enacted legislation around the world. The Environmental Health Trust team is engaged in educating legislators at the local, state, provincial, and federal level in North America and advocating on behalf of impacted communities around the world. First and foremost, EHT is unique in its focus on conducting and evaluating key research on this topic and others that address environmental exposures to plants, animals, and humans.

While we may not have all the answers yet, *Disconnect* gives an in-depth understanding of why these government agencies are not responding. The website for Environmental Health Trust and others noted in the expanded section on resources in this new edition provide extensive information on why and how to advance safer technologies.

C4ST does similar education, awareness, and advocacy work to EHT. We are among many organizations globally that are picking up the mantle and organizing to raise the alarms and protect humans, wildlife, and the environment from the unchecked rollout of 5G and beyond. When you read *Disconnect*, my expectation is that you too will become concerned about the tech and telecom industries' plans to deploy the Internet of Things powered by 5G without any effort to limit exposures.

During these challenging times, it is tempting to dismiss the concerns we are raising about electromagnetic fields as unimportant, given the rife conflicts the world faces. On the contrary, now is precisely the moment in human history when we must focus our efforts on protecting our children from these pervasive invisible hazards on which we are excessively dependent. We should not allow ourselves to let convenience trump our health or our planet.

We are at a critical turning point. If our government agencies do not step up to expedite substantial improvements in our safety regulations, shift toward the installation of fiber optic cable to and through our schools, workplaces, and homes, and hold the technology and telecommunications industries accountable for their reckless disregard of public health, it may be too late. Fortunately, this new edition of *Disconnect* offers additional guidance on why and how to go about reducing or limiting your exposure as we wait for our government agencies and the private sector to do the right thing. You may not be able to depend on them, but you can count on *Disconnect* to steer you toward safety. We should all heed its advice.

AUTHOR'S INTRODUCTION, 2024

T he global conversation around cell phones and other wireless radiating devices has shifted radically since the first edition of *Disconnect* in 2010. What had been a bare whisper has become a resounding roar. Evidence regarding the damaging impacts of radiation on our health and that of the world around us has become irrefutable.

The response to these concerns? Just as described in our first edition, a well-funded manufacturing of doubt is now recognized as the worldwide strategy to undermine both the science and the scientists. Framing the issue as highly uncertain and complicated prolongs confusion and inaction.

Just because the issue of microwave radiation is complex does not mean that people are incapable of understanding the need to reduce exposure. Keeping two-way microwave radiating and receiving devices close to the body is ill-advised. As evidence of the harmful psychological and physical impact grows, many developed nations now ban or severely limit cell phones in schools and set limits for exposures that are up to 1,000 times lower than those of the U.S., Canada, and Australia.

France has been especially fertile territory for actions to reduce exposures, reflecting in some part the valiant efforts to encourage government actions by scientists like my former colleague, the best-selling author and neuroscientist, David Servan-Schreiber, MD, PhD, who died of a brain tumor, and physician-epidemiologist Annie Sasco MD, DSc, as well as dozens of other scientists and engineers. Goaded by physician Marc Arazi and our colleagues with Phone-gate Alerte in France, the French government released data in 2018 confirming that 9 out of 10 phones — out of more than 400 phones on the market — failed to comply with its own obsolete standards by as much as fourfold. Several million phones have been recalled as a result. No such monitoring or review of phone radiation occurs in the U.S. or Canada, where outdated permitted exposures are the highest in the world. Nor is there any posting of real-time exposures from the more than one million wireless-radiating network coverage antennas currently used in those nations. Standing apart from many other countries, in September of 2023, the French government banned sales of the iPhone 12 due to its excessive radiation as measured with outdated safety standards based solely on avoiding heating. Other governments are also taking some actions, begging the question of why and how nations can rely on such outmoded ways of measuring this type of electromagnetic radiation in the first place.

It is easy to understand how interjecting confusion has become the working strategy, part of what industry public relations mavens literally dubbed "war-games." In fact, the application of a variety of electromagnetic (EMF) devices in medicine — dubbed electroceuticals — offers an expanding range of clinical options that employ EMF from bone healing to treatment of chronic depression and cancer. As with all drugs, any agent that can heal can also be damaging depending on how, when, and where it is used. Thus, it should not be surprising to learn that there indeed can be a dark side to the biological impacts of electromagnetic radiation.

In 2011 — just one year after the publication of *Disconnect* — an expert review panel of the World Health Organization's International Agency for Research on Cancer (WHO/IARC) produced highly inconvenient science: it declared the radio frequency EMF emissions from cell phones and other electronic sources a "possible human carcinogen" — the same category as DDT and chloroform. They reached this conclusion after reviewing all relevant experimental and epidemiological evidence. The IARC is now under concerted attack to reverse its determination, as industry manufactures doubts about the science, bolstered by the official sounding International Commission on Non-Ionizing Radiation Protection (ICNIRP). Despite its close ties with industry and lack of transparency, a number of governments rely on ICNIRP declarations when crafting policy.

Fortunately, highly informed, independent experts' efforts have emerged that are producing a much-needed counterweight to ICNIRP. Statements of concern and specific recommendations about why and how to reduce exposures have been advanced by the American Academy of Pediatrics (APP), the Oceania Radiofrequency Scientific Advisory Association (ORSAA), a non-profit independent group of former government advisors and radiation experts from South Asia and Australia; the International Commission on Biological Effects of EMF (ICBE-EMF), a consortium of multidisciplinary experts producing paradigm-busting publications on why and how to make wireless technology safer; the BabySafe Project, a group of more than 400 physicians and expert researchers formed by Grassroots Environmental Education and Environmental Health Trust; Physicians for Safe Technology, and a growing number of others. These independent groups stand in stark contrast to ICNIRP and its insouciant recommendations.

In 2007, Sasco, Servan-Schreiber, Ronald B. Herberman MD, the inspiring founder of the University of Pittsburgh's Cancer Institute, and I issued a broad call for research and precaution in the use of mobile devices. This call was signed by dozens of medical and bio-electromagnetic experts. Since then a growing number of other expert groups have developed detailed appeals for preventive policies that reduce exposures while increasing research. In Australia and New Zealand, ORSAA expressly noted the need to update standards in Australia, Canada, and the U.S. Most recently, our colleagues from down under resoundingly declared that the assumption that 5G is safe does not rest on scientific evidence. These developments make clear that the absence of definitive proof of harm is not evidence of safety.

One year after the WHO/IARC's 2011 declaration placed cell phone radiation in the same category as chloroform — a suspected human carcinogen — Professor John Wargo of Yale University issued a report for the Environment and Human Health Institute affirming the need to take precautionary steps to reduce cell phone exposures especially in light of growing exposures to children. In innovative experiments, Professor Hugh Taylor, Chief of Obstetrics and Gynecology at Yale Medical Center, showed that prenatally exposed rodents developed offspring with shortened attention spans and serious behavioral problems. A series of studies produced by the NATO-sponsored laboratories of Nesrin Seyhan of Gazi University in Ankara and Suleyman Kaplan of Ondokuz Mayis University in Samsun, Turkey, have documented reduced brain size and more brain damage in prenatally exposed rats, rabbits, and mice.

In 2018, following the most extended and intense review accorded one of its reports since its founding 40 years earlier, the U.S. National Toxicology Program (NTP) produced state-of-the-art experimental studies confirming that current levels of cell phone radiation create very rare, highly malignant tumors of the brain in tested rodents. Other publications from the NTP confirm that this same radiation can damage DNA in several different organs—a hallmark of agents that can cause cancer or neurological damage. Shortly thereafter, the acclaimed Ramazzini Institute issued similar findings. While we differ in many fortunate ways from other animals, we humans are not that different. We share most of their DNA. Every agent found to cause cancer in animals also produces it in humans when adequately studied, according to the IARC.

As my mentor, Mount Sinai Medical Center Professor Irving Selikoff, often reminded us, public health statistics are human beings with the tears removed. I've been a numbers person most of my professional life. As a trained epidemiologist and toxicologist, I discern patterns created by illnesses and deaths of sufficient numbers of humans, animals, or cultures of their cells.

At its core, epidemiology must operate by counting and evaluating patterns in time and space that deaths or illnesses comprise in an effort to tease out the origins of disease or study remedies. The bane of my life is the "N of one" — where there are only one or two cases with a particular health outcome and suspected exposures. Not everything of importance can be arrayed in ways that achieve what is deemed to be significant. Sometimes a well-conducted clinical evaluation of a single case report can change the face of medicine. This happened when mid-twentieth century reports showed that in a few cases, a cardiac catheter could safely be inserted into the heart to measure blood flow or blockages. This thoroughly reported astonishing development spawned the life-saving field of interventional cardiology.

To make sense of mounting relevant statistics, I have worked with a number of brilliant minds, including one of the world's leading cancer epidemiologists, Professor Emeritus of Epidemiology, Anthony B. Miller, who has published more than 600 peer-reviewed articles and frequently advised the World Health Organization. Looking at all the human and animal studies amassed as of 2019, nearly a decade *after* the publication of *Disconnect,* Miller and I concluded that the grounds linking wireless radiation and cancer had become stronger and can no longer be ignored. Especially worrisome are findings from Sweden that those who began using cell phones regularly as teenagers have four to eight times more malignant glioma as adults. In fact, cell phone-like radiation speeds up the growth of thyroid and rectal cancer cells and also damages fast-growing sperm.

The causes for the puzzling fourfold increases in colo-rectal cancer in persons under age forty since 2010 in the U.S. and many other industrialized nations may be traceable to the habit of keeping wireless radiating phones on and in the pocket or tucked directly over the lower body. Experimental studies show that this radiation accelerates the growth of colo-rectal cancer cells under controlled conditions. Coupled with the fact that phones are tested at some distance off the body, surely this evidence of the susceptibility of colo-rectal cancer to wireless phone radiation strengthens the case for reducing this exposure at this time.

Of course, one cannot definitively say what underlies these trends. As Albert Einstein once put it, "Not everything that counts can be counted and not everything that can be counted counts."

That's where laboratory studies can be quite useful. Remember — every agent that causes cancer in humans also produces it in animals when adequately studied. Thus, the absence of overall increased trends in cancer in the general population should not be misconstrued as proof of phone safety. The technology is too new, the expanded uses too recent, and the ways we employ phones keep changing, making it even more challenging to evaluate their impacts. We have so little data because it's challenging to study the issue and little funding or training goes to advancing our understanding."

In fact, cancer typically has a long latency or period of time from when important exposures begin and the disease becomes evident. The expected latency for relatively rare cancers of the brain is four or five decades. About 60 percent of all brain cancers are glioblastoma, most of which occur in persons aged 65 and older. The elderly have not been heavy users of cell phones historically. When you look more closely at what's happening with younger persons, some unexplained increases in cancer are evident, including rises in rates of glioma and thyroid cancer reported by the Centers for Disease Control and Prevention. While diagnostic improvements may partly account for the growth in thyroid cancer, that certainly cannot explain all the recent upticks in young people, including the colo-rectal cancer rates in the under-forty cohort.

Responding to the new science indicating the need to reduce exposures, and so far resisting industry entreaties, more than a dozen high-tech nations have developed policies to reduce wireless radiation, especially around children, requiring that phones be sold with headsets and information about why and how to keep them and other wireless radiating devices off the body. Some may recall that the first BlackBerry phones came with leather cases and advice not to use them next to the brain or belly. When those notices no longer appeared, the implication many drew was that whatever issue may have once been relevant had become irrelevant. Not so. Instead, the industry simply moved notices to keep phones off the body from fine print warnings in flimsy pamphlets easily tossed away to deep within their operating systems.

Sometime shortly after *Disconnect* was published with its call to read fine print packaging, Apple responded. It stopped issuing package-printed guidance altogether. Advice about tested distance was moved to inside the phone for access — provided you know how and where to look for it. Simply go to settings>general>about>legal>rf exposure and there you will find the notice: to avoid exceeding the tested exposure limits, use a headset or speakerphone and do not keep the phone on the body.

Few are generally aware that under Federal Communications Commission (FCC) requirements manufacturers select a unit of each phone model to be tested at some distance from the body and brain with a "spacer" of 10 millimeters or more to allow for the ear. Every single millimeter away from the body means 15 percent less exposure, according to University of Utah Professor Emeritus Om Gandhi, a pioneer of the field of bioelectromagnetics.

We live in perverse times where phones are regularly advertised featuring playful toddlers and media-obsessed teens using devices in ways that far exceed the FCC's outdated test limits and in precisely the ways that the fine print warnings advise against. Thousands of apps can be downloaded for infants and toddlers, whose fast-growing brains quickly become addicted to digital toys that become preferred over simple human contact. Few know or heed the American Academy of Pediatrics' caution that young children be limited in screen time and that families not allow devices at the table during meals.

Since March 2014 in Belgium, it has been against the law to sell baby button cell phones marketed to children age seven and younger. In Taiwan, as of April 2015, giving a phone to a child age two or younger is a crime. In Israel and India, teachers are forbidden from requiring classroom use of cell phones. In Turkey, ads to and with children using phones have been outlawed since 2011. Many nations ban or severely limit phones in schools as evidence of their harmful psychological and physical impacts grows.

Several independent investigations, from the Canadian Broadcasting Corporation (CBC) to the *Chicago Sun-Times,* have confirmed what *Disconnect* noted in 2010 and what our French collaborators have established — when phones are used against the body, they exceed the test limits established by the U.S. government in 1996 and still in force today. For CBC's *Marketplace,* investigative journalist Wendy Mesley showed in 2017 that when phones were tested next to the body — rather than with the rigged system currently in place — they could exceed current outdated standards four- to five-fold. Although that same result — originally foretold in *Disconnect* — was corroborated independently by the *Chicago Sun-Times* in 2019, those facts faded quickly from public discourse. Mesley's extraordinary reporting and coverage by neurosurgeon-journalist Sanjay Gupta for CNN on electromagnetic fields had spectacular but very short shelf lives.

Meanwhile, pathological attachment to devices has become a classified mental health diagnosis, as has FOMO, the "fear of missing out," that keeps many chained to their devices from the bedroom to the bathroom and beyond. Apps teaching toddlers to use the potty have resulted in youngsters being unable to use the toilet without a screen. It has not escaped public attention that several mass shooters spent much of their disturbed, mentally ill lives mired in hate-mongering social media. In Asia, camps have been created to treat children as young as eight who have become addicted to gaming and screens.

Global declines in school performance provide a worrying signal that this may be partly linked to the over-reliance on digital devices, especially when used by young children. In the U.S., as evidence of ever-younger eZombies mounts, a growing number of experts, teachers, parents, community health advocates, documentary filmmakers, and grandparents are becoming educated and motivated about why and how to reduce exposure to wireless devices for the sake of our mental and physical health.

Life is not an ongoing emergency, although increasingly more and more devices suited for disaster communications intrude into personal spaces, dinner tables, playgrounds, bedrooms and bathrooms, where their always-on components can corrupt in-person social dynamics. Toddlers of parents who are heavy device users have delays in learning to talk. As Sophia Ruan Gushée has noted on her website (Ruanliving.com), technology can create breakdowns in communication within families. Psychologists have coined the term "technoference" to indicate when technologies disrupt basic human relationships, especially those of parent-to-child or romantic partners. The phrase 'absent presence' designates being physically present but preoccupied with technological signals, noises, likes, links, and other updates. Some obsessive behaviors with technology are now listed as certified psychiatric disorders under the Diagnostic and Statistical Manual of Mental Disorders (DSM).

Highly regarded medical experts like New York Times best-selling author, Mark Hyman, MD, are issuing practical advice to lessen radiation exposures and dependencies. Psychiatrist Victoria Dunckley ensures harried parents that setting digital limits sets the stage for healthier families. There is now increasing acknowledgment that wireless radiation constitutes a serious problem that could, in part, account for unexplained increases or worsening of a plethora of health problems — autism, ADHD, chronic fatigue syndrome, multiple sclerosis, diabetes, Parkinson's, and Alzheimer's, to name a few.

The same year that the WHO/IARC declared radio frequency electromagnetic fields a possible carcinogen, the former president of Microsoft Canada, Frank Clegg — a thirty-year veteran in the telecom and computer industry — founded the nonprofit consumer advocacy group, Canadians for Safe Technology (C4ST), to promote sensible policies regarding cell phones and other wireless transmitting devices. R. Blank, a successful technology innovator, multi-talented author, programmer, and cutting-edge designer for Microsoft, Google, and Apple, created Shield Your Body, a company making patches that block microwave radiation. When Robert Szcerba, a former Lockheed Martin rocket scientist, corporate director of Global Healthcare and Life Sciences, self-described technology geek, and a prolific blogger at Forbes.com, began asking uncomfortable questions about the safety of Wi-Fi for children, this unleashed a firestorm of responses.

Scientific evidence on cell phone harms is also fueling important advances in legal actions worldwide. A man who developed a disabling tumor from using his cell phone was awarded compensation by an Italian court in 2019. Workers in Austria can now be covered for such injuries as well. Closer to home, in the U.S. Superior Court of the District of Columbia in Washington, D.C., Judge Frederick Weissberg has ruled that there is sufficient legal and scientific merit for men with malignant brain tumors to seek damages from telecom firms and manufacturers for causing their illnesses.

Case closed? Nope. Unsurprisingly, their case remains in legal limbo, which may not be resolved for some time. Several nations are taking a closer look at ways to protect their citizens. Most remain blithely unaware that phones, tablets, and other devices include advisories to keep off the body. Innovative businesses are offering a variety of tools to keep phones away from the body. The independent start-up Green Swan in 2014 produced an app that flashed warnings whenever a device was held closer than outdated guidelines. In 2016, Samsung marketed a quite similar app that flashed warnings when it detected a face that was "too close." When given a chance to install the Tawkon app to automatically flash red, orange, or blue indicators of safety inside the early generation of iPhone in 2008, Steve Jobs replied to its former Israeli intelligence developers, "Not interested." Amazingly, in 2023, Apple added a similar warning system to iOS17 phones to alert users against eye strain and myopia.

Although they may well deflect radiation to other body parts, stick-on fabrics that block radiation can be ironed into pants pockets and are selling well in some geek quarters.

Among their biggest customers? The young and not-so-young technorati, who are also grabbing soft radiation-blocking shawls or blankets to be draped over pregnant bellies. From Silicon Valley, California, to Korea, men who want to father healthy children are also using these radiation blocking fabrics. In Korea, China, and other Asian nations, one of the first signs of pregnancy occurs when a woman sports a belly radiation shield made of soft-metal embedded fabric that can be ordered on Asian Ebay-like websites.

Digital detox retreats and products are flourishing among social media mavens. Arianna Huffington warns of her own digital burnout. Former elite fashion model Shannon Vaughan has started Pursoma—a company dedicated to products that enhance recovery from chemical and other toxic exposures. Gwyneth Paltrow's Goop promotes life less harried. Jess Davis, founder of folkrebellion.com, spurs efforts to avoid digital meltdowns and wrest control of parenting from digital trolls.

There is an increasing awareness among the public with regards to the dangers of cell phone radiation. Increasing numbers of people refuse to put cell phones next to their heads and use headphones or speaker phones to talk. Many schools have taken the step to ban the use of cell phones by students and rely on wired rather than wireless for all forms of computer use.

Determined to stop the spread of phones into elementary schools, a number of parents are signing on to "wait until eighth"— supporting parents to resist social pressures. In fact, Korean psychiatrists have diagnosed digital dementia in middle-schoolers addicted to gaming. Teens that use phones regularly have impaired memory according to replicated Swiss studies. What makes all this especially disconcerting is that animal studies have predicted precisely these results. In 2015, Indian researchers concluded that rats exposed during pregnancy to cell phone radiation developed damage to their brain DNA and significant deficits in learning, essentially replicating studies from researchers in Yale Professor Taylor's lab.

The BabySafe Project, a joint initiative of more than three hundred of the world's top physicians, scientists, and educators in public health, including Yale's Professor Taylor, was founded in 2015 to inform women and their physicians about the risk two-way microwave wireless radiation from cell phones poses to pregnancy and to urge expectant mothers to limit their exposures. Already, they have handed out millions of advisories to pregnant women in the U.S., India, South Africa, Turkey, Colombia, Canada, Israel, and many other nations.

In 2022 the nonpartisan New Hampshire Commission on 5G assessed the science thoroughly (detailed in the last chapter of this book). Kent Chamberlin, Past Chair and Professor Emeritus of Electrical and Computer Engineering of the University of New Hampshire, has spent his career studying how electromagnetic radiation affects devices and the human body and holds patents on antenna design. A leader of the New Hampshire Commission on 5G, and a founding member of the ICBE-EMF, he is one of the hundreds of experts speaking out about growing concerns that we cannot continue to rely on twentieth century standards to test twenty-first century technology. In numerous presentations in North America and abroad, Chamberlin is advising that cell phone radiation, including 5G, poses a significant threat to human health and the environment. Along with other leaders of the ICBE-EMF, he believes that antennas should be especially configured to reduce what falls within their wireless plumes and that no source of microwave radiation should be located within 500 meters of places where people live or work. Environmental Health Trust, the organization I have led for more than 15 years, heartily agrees.

Sadly, the list of scientific pioneers on the damaging impacts of wireless radiation who are no longer with us, including, notably, Martin Blank, is growing. Blank's book, *Overpowered,* confirmed and expanded on his decades of basic research detailing how low levels of electromagnetic fields could impede the basic functioning of living cells. Herberman and Maryann Donovan — my deputy director at the Center for Environmental Oncology at the University of Pittsburgh's Cancer Institute — both died far too young. Along with other Pitt colleagues, they steadfastly encouraged and supported the formation of EHT — which has carried forward their concerns. Herberman and Donovan would be pleased with the progress. Doktor Professor Franz Adlkofer, profiled here in 2010 for persisting in publishing highly inconvenient findings that phone radiation directly damaged the DNA of the brain, died in 2022 on his beloved island of Paros. Before his death, he prevailed in his decade-long effort to have German courts compel those who challenged his scientific credibility to recant and cease their defamatory critiques. Invited by Professor Lawrence Lessig, Adlkofer and I participated in a Harvard Law School seminar on ethics that highlighted his valiant efforts.

For me one loss hits especially hard — my dear friend, the brilliant young neuropsychiatrist David Servan-Schreiber. His book, *Anticancer*, published in 2007, constituted a veritable breakthrough — a sensitive, thoughtful explanation of his efforts against cancer as a young scientist. Featured on public television and translated into 40 languages, he crafted the scientific foundations for advancing nutrition and lifestyle practices to reduce the chances that cancer can occur or recur, keeping his own early brain cancer in abeyance. In the first preface to *Disconnect*, he explained that until the moment we met in 2007 (when he was 47), it had not dawned on him that placing a microwave radiating device next to his head for hours a day for more than a decade might promote a resurgence of cancer. After looking at the studies Sasco, Herberman, Donovan, and I had amassed, he never again put a phone to his head. It was too late. Prophetically, he wrote in the first foreword to *Disconnect*:

> "We don't want to believe that our new toys to which we are so attached — and which bring in enormous profits — could also cause our demise or that of our children. But science is not about belief. The government's responsibility to its citizens should not be either."

In that same note, Servan-Schreiber pointedly observed that insurance companies refused to cover cell phone companies and operators in case of claims of health damage from long-term operation of their devices, a fact that remains true to this day. The worldwide multi-trillion dollar telecommunications industry remains self-insured. During the last decade several global secondary insurance firms compared the risks of covering damages from electromagnetic radiation to those of asbestos — a problem that bankrupted many companies that faced billions in claims. In 2019, Swiss Re, a global multi-billion dollar business, declared the risks of insuring 5G to be "off the leash," meaning out of control and similar to those of asbestos.

Within two years of penning his words of warning, at the too-young age of fifty, Servan-Schreiber was dead from a massive brain cancer. As his close friend and colleague, I am confident that he would have been pleased that in 2021, the U.S. Circuit Court of Appeals for the District of Columbia ruled in a landmark case brought by Environmental Health Trust and others that the FCC had not provided proof that it had read the thousands of pages of submitted scientific evidence since the FCC's safety limits were first issued in 1996, including reports from Servan-Schreiber and dozens of others. The court termed the refusal to update the last-century limits "arbitrary and capricious." It observed that the FCC ignored evidence on children's vulnerability, consequences of long-term exposure, damage to memory and sperm, environmental impacts (to birds, bees, trees, etc), along with testimony from hundreds of individuals documenting a wide range of injuries, including electro hypersensitivity — exquisite physiological reactions to EMF."

Some two years after the nation's second highest court told the FCC to review its outdated standards for testing phones, the agency has not responded. Thus, the FCC's 1996 limits do not rest on an up-to-date scientific review. Rather they reflect the phenomenal grip that industry has on the agency, as noted by Norm Alster in his 2015 report issued by Harvard's Safra Center for Ethics that dubbed the FCC "a captured agency." A letter to the agency from Wyoming Governor Mark Gordon wanting to know how it plans to address this glaring problem of outmoded standards also remains unanswered.

Think about it. Government regulators rely on 1996 safety standards to back industry claims that current technology is safe. Would you want to use 1996 lead paint standards? Not until 2009 were lead paint standards established in 1977 lowered more than sixfold from

600 to 90 ppm. Would you want to fly in an airplane with 1996 standards of safety? After federal goals mandated improved safety standards in 1996, the same year safety standards were set for cell phones, deaths from airplane crashes dropped by more than half. These are remarkable demonstrations of government and industry working for the benefit of the public. Yet no such cooperation is in the offing to improve the 1996 standards for cellular radiation.

James C. Lin is a Professor Emeritus at the University of Illinois, a former commissioner of ICNIRP, Life Fellow of the Institute of Electrical and Electronics Engineers, and former Editor-in-Chief of *Bioelectromagnetics* — a vital journal in the field. In a series of publications over the past several years, he has deemed current safety limits irrelevant, debatable, and without scientific foundation, concluding that there is little substance underlying the ongoing 5G rollout. As this book was going to press in December 2023, Lin wrote an essay for *IEEE Microwave Magazine* describing what might turn out to be a seismic shift. Since 2017, the U.S. Department of Defense has been funding research into nonthermal impacts of radio frequency radiation. These studies directly contradict the ICNIRP insistence that no such effects exist. Additionally, current limits ignore important animal and modeling data, especially regarding 5G, for which there are no adequate health studies. Lin concludes, "Many of the recommended limits are questionable from the standpoint of scientific justification for the safety and public health protection."

Environmental Health Trust continues to champion critically important research clarifying the nature of the risks from wireless radiation and proposing several simple solutions for reducing those risks in homes, schools, and workplaces. For the past decade, I have been joined in this enterprise by our relentless and fiercely determined Executive Director, Theodora Scarato, who had been compelled to move her children to a school that would provide reduced radiation.

What can you do now? Share this book with your friends and family. Make sure they appreciate that the science has become clearer. Work with Environmental Health Trust and your local libraries to see that book clubs assign this new edition. For the first 50 public libraries that ask to form discussion programs, EHT will make a dozen copies of *Disconnect* available at no charge, along with a guide for community conversations with students, parents, teachers, and local officials. EHT can help provide simple testing meters that can be placed on library loan so that people can learn how to make crude measures of exposures. Check out and share the practical advice offered in chapter 15 of this new edition about simple ways that you can reduce your exposures.

Help us help you develop simple ways to reduce direct radiation for yourselves and your children by linking to our website, ehtrust. org, for more information on why and how to reduce your exposures.

We are with phones today where we were with cars in the 1960s. We need the equivalent of airbags and seat belts for our wireless mobile devices. The technology exists. Industry understands that people are waking up to the simple fact that this technology can and must be made more safe. Cell phones are not toys, as manufacturers' inserts from several companies noted more than a decade ago. We know that they can be made safer through simple changes in hardware and software, tapping existing patents, and using devices in ways described in chapter 15 of this edition and on EHT's website.

Wise social critic Margaret Mead once noted: "Never doubt that a small group of thoughtful, committed citizens can change the world; indeed, it's the only thing that ever has."

-Devra Davis, PhD, MPH, 2024

1

KIDS, WE'LL GET BACK TO YOU

Kids, We'll Get Back To You

Who can protest and does not is an accomplice in the act.

~ Talmud

Could cell phones be unsafe? When I first heard this idea about six years ago, I did not believe it and I did not want to believe it. I had been an early and enthusiastic adopter of this revolutionary technology, which I put to good use managing a staff of several dozen scientists in two different buildings at the National Academy of Sciences. I used it to stay in touch with my children and husband at odd times and places. I prided myself on being able to keep up with my grad students on the latest geeky applications. I knew that most scientists were convinced it was simply impossible for radio frequency radiation from phones to have any impact on human biology. But, as someone who has spent my entire professional career examining the links between the environment and health, I realized that, like the rest of us, science and scientists follow fads and fashions. Sometimes what everyone wants to believe turns out to be inconveniently wrong. Authorities in technologically sophisticated nations, like Israel and

29

Finland, where phones had been used longer and more heavily, had issued warnings about safer use of phones. I began to ask why.

In this book I present what I found. It astonished me. And it still does. I hope by the time you finish reading this book, you will share my view — and those of growing numbers of experts in this country and abroad — that we would be foolish to not take simple precautions. Cell phone designs can and probably will be improved to lower direct exposures to the brain and body. But, in the meantime, we can reduce radio frequency radiation from cell phones, while science pursues the matter fully — something it has not yet done.

Contrary to the firmly held beliefs of many respected authorities, invisible radio frequency radiation can alter living cells and create the same types of damage that we know increase the risk of cancer and neurological disease. Neither the danger nor the safety of cell phones is yet certain. How we manage that uncertainty could avert a global public health catastrophe.

Each one of our world's six-plus billion people starts life with a brain that is not fully formed. With luck and decent nutrition, by the time we hit our early twenties our brains have become completely "wired." By the time you are reading this book there will be about five billion cell phones on this planet. You may even own two of them. And you almost certainly know many people with growing brains (anyone under twenty-five) who regularly use cell phones. Children are growing up in a swamp of radio frequency radiation that did not exist even five years ago.

Cell phones have revolutionized our ability to respond to emergencies real and imagined. They provide social status. They help you find a job. They neatly store all the music you want to listen to and summon up loved ones anytime, anywhere. They seem essential to connecting you with whatever you want to do: track stocks, share favorite photos, download sports results, and send text, images, videos, and voice notes throughout the global village. To succeed you need to be reachable 24/7. And who can argue that these wonderful gadgets do make you feel more in touch, more effective, more, well, fun? The newest generation of phones brings us closer, faster, and nearer to one another than ever before.

Cell phones today are like electricity and water — things we can't live without. They seem so benign and so invaluable. Cell phones are used to call ambulances but are never the reason for the call in the first place. Yet we have overlooked something — something more insidious than the dangers of texting while driving. There is a disconnect between the way that cell phones tie us all together and what these revolutionary tools can do to our bodies as they press up against our ears every day.

I'm probably a tenth generation "bubbie," the Yiddish word for grandmother. Actually my own mother liked to be called by the American moniker Grandma Jean. But, in fact, she came, like me, from a long line of bubbies: Bubbie Fannie, Bubbie Pearl, Bubbie Leah. Just like all grandmothers in the world, I want to keep my grandchildren safe.

My grandkids come equipped with an array of modern protective armor. They have their own car seats and bike helmets and know all about the need to buckle up. My eldest grandchild, Davis, nearly five, wears a white plastic helmet sitting tightly over his dark brown curly hair, and black Velcro pads for wrists, knees, and elbows, whenever he rides his skateboard. He is a grandmother's delight in blue jeans and a red checkered shirt swooshing down the sidewalk by Capitol Hill (excellent skateboarding terrain close to our home). Davis is all concentration, as he waits until the walk is clear. He heads pell-mell straight down the middle of the pavement, stops the board abruptly by stepping down hard on the back edge, makes it pop right up in the air, then proudly hops off usually without falling.

I actually have a hard time walking as fast as he can ride. Just over three feet tall, Davis rules the sidewalk, just as long as his sister Josephine, a mere eighteen months younger and six inches shorter, lets him. Curly-brown-haired Josephine proudly pedals her tricycle as fast as she can, tongue sticking out. Her helmet is shimmery pink as she pedals right at her older brother, Davis, but she stops short. Jo Jo has already perfected that second child victim pout. She's about to whine.

Watching my two young grandchildren at play as they jockey for position on the sidewalk, I can almost hear the neurons firing. The difference between being alive and being dead is just one thing — the presence of electrical activity in the brain. Josephine and Davis know they are being watched. They glance plaintively to me, hoping I will intervene. We decide to go inside and see a new family toy.

Their dad has brought home a small plastic box that is a bit big for their little hands, with a screen that rotates images. Josephine and Davis are enchanted. They each want that Droid — the spanking new phone, the one that plays music, shows cartoons and videos, talks, and tells Dad where to drive and find an open store for soft-serve ice cream.

They've grown up with tranquilizing DVDs beamed into the family van. Now here is a little screen that does all that and a whole lot more.

Our brain controls what we see, think, feel, hear — how we sense the world around us. By the second month of prenatal life, a simple cylinder of nerve cells forms in the center of the growing embryo. From this hollow tube the human brain grows at the incredible speed of a quarter million cells a minute, going from zero to one hundred billion cells at birth. The brain of an infant triples in weight in the first year of life and doubles to two hundred billion cells by the age of two. There are so many connections among these cells that it would take more than thirty million years merely to count them aloud. With each signal my toddler grandchildren take in, the rods and cones in their eyes dart to whatever most catches their fancy, their ears tune in to the sounds striking their auditory nerves, and their center of wants — the amygdala — presses them onward to demand whatever it is they decide they must have or do.

Infants cannot focus their eyes, but they can and do attune to patterns and smells that attract their brains. By the time they are a few months old, babies can see and sense their moms and dads. Their brains settle in to regular rhythms to sleep, to eat, to cry, and do it all over again as they grow. Each one of those billions of cells they are born with can be connected to half a dozen others. Infant brains are like small supercomputers, with hard-to-grasp numbers of combinations and permutations inside their soft skulls.

What about that phone they are each set to have? What explains its nearly hypnotic power for those tender minds? My grandkids are enthralled by the small, shiny new black Droid. But it might be an iPhone or a Palm Pre. The American Academy of Pediatrics advises strongly that parents not rely on television and videos to calm babies. But try telling that to the harried mother of three in diapers. Kids become enthralled, seemingly powerless to resist. Evolution clearly didn't prepare them for this. Nothing so brilliantly colored and musical, so fluctuating and wild, so exquisitely scaled, existed out there on the African savannah a million years ago. Davis figured out how to play the common cell phone game *BrickBreaker* before he could read or count. These new toys can be utterly irresistible. Children have always loved to pretend-talk on phones. So why shouldn't a kindergartener be able to chatter to his grandparents on the phone, now that he or she can, anywhere, anytime, quite conveniently? The games, Internet access, global positioning information — what's the problem with all these interesting treats? Why not give all toddlers a cell phone? The reason is that there is a disconnect between what the scientific world knows about cell phone radiation and the benign reputation these slick gadgets have.

If we could take a slow motion movie of the growth of the brain, we would see that the master computer leading its development spins faster than any mortal can count and it does not sit in a superhero Iron Man case. Unlike a metal shelled machine, the skull of a child is very soft. This is a good thing, as it means that when curious playful infants fall, as they have been doing for millions of years, their heads are less likely to break. A baby's cranium is made of thin bone that continues to grow and ultimately becomes thicker. The faster that any cells are growing, the greater the chance they can make mistakes and endlessly repeat them. The thinner and pliant skulls of children help them survive, as evolution designed, but the lack of 3G cell phones on the African savannah millions of years ago has left children susceptible to the radiation these phones now emit.

Try saying a tongue twister slowly — *Peter Piper picked a peck of pickled peppers. How many pecks of pickled peppers did Peter Piper pick?* Now say it again faster. Then say it as fast as you can. With any increase in speed will come more mistakes. The brain of a three-year-old weighs three-fourths as much as that of an adult and gobbles up twice as much blood sugar. The young brain continues to grow throughout childhood and adolescence. It's not just the sheer number of brain cells or neurons that increase, it's also the ways that they are connected to one another. Over time, fatty coatings of myelin surround neurons, giving them more strength and resilience. This protective coating is much more than window dressing. Myelin is believed to confer judgment, wisdom, impulse control, and many other properties we associate with maturity and a good life. It will not surprise parents who have survived teenage drivers in the family to learn that the human brain does not fully mature until the twenties. That this maturation happens a bit later for young men than young women — also no surprise to many parents.

As with any other developing tissue the brain is vulnerable to toxic exposures, especially if they occur early on. Infinitesimal amounts of the heavy metal lead encountered in the first two years of life can lead to a host of nasty neural consequences. Lead has a computible number of electrons surrounding its atoms as calcium. This means that this toxic metal competes with and can block calcium from being taken into the brain and other vital parts of the body. Calcium is essential for brain and bone health and for our heartbeats and neurons. Lead is not only not needed, it has the ability to throw microscopic monkey wrenches into neurons and synapses, if it gets a chance. Children with just a bit too much lead and too little calcium in the first years of life end up with lower intelligence, more problems in school, and ultimately tend to find their ways into jails and mental institutions at much greater rates as young adults.

If toddlers exposed to lead develop permanently diminished brains and more criminal and psychiatric problems as adults, how will their minds and bodies be affected by the unprecedented flood of radio frequency signals in which they are growing up today? In the years after World War II, encouraged by the sudden availability and enthusiasm for military surplus technology, doctors thought it made sense to use X-rays to treat ringworm — an infectious disease of the scalp. It worked. The X-rays cleaned up the infection, but they also left a much more toxic legacy. Children whose brains were irradiated for a short period of time to treat scalp infections before age five develop almost four times more brain tumors by the time they reach middle age than those who didn't go through such treatments.

The brain of a child needs all the protection it can get as early and for as long as possible. The helmets my grandson and his sisters wear keep their skulls from getting cracked by sudden falls, but they do nothing to stop the absorption of small microwave signals into their brains that come from phones. Phones today are smaller, smarter, and faster than ever before. Are they as benign as they seem?

In 2000, the former prime minister of Norway, Gro Harlem Brundtland, a physician, became director general of the World Health Organization (WHO), the world's premiere public health agency. Trained at the Harvard School of Public Health, Brundtland headed the United Nations Commission on Sustainable Development. In 2002, she sat down with a reporter from a leading Norwegian newspaper and revealed that she had banned cell phones from her office at the WHO. During the course of the interview, she began to get a headache. Brundtland asked whether someone in the room might have a cell phone that was on. The newspaper's photographer had turned his ringer off but left his phone on, figuring that Brundtland would never know he had done so. He was wrong.

Brundtland was embarrassed by her physical reaction. But it was a problem she could not ignore.

"I made several tests: People have been in my office with their mobile hidden in their pocket or bag. Without knowing if it was on or off. I have always reacted when the phone has been on — never when it's off. So . . ."

She did not advise people against using a mobile phone at the time; as a physician, she believed that scientific research had not made the case for offering such advice. Brundtland said that she expected that the world would soon have important information about the long-term impact of cell phones. "At this time we do not have scientific evidence to go out with a clear warning. It is not established that the radiation, for instance, can result in brain cancer. WHO has a big study going on and in two or three years from now, we will have better answers to all these questions." In other words, "We'll get back to you."

In fact it took more than eight years for that study to be released. The official verdict is that "biases and errors limit the strength of the conclusions that can be drawn." They advise that "further investigation of mobile phone use and brain cancer risk is merited."

This scenario begins to reveal why there is such an extraordinary disconnect between what scientists have come to learn in the last few years, building on little known research that is now decades old, and the miraculous, unquestioned, and benign aura of today's smart phones. This book is about that disconnect.

2

HOW THE FIRES OF
TECHNOLOGY SHOCK AND AWE

The Lord giveth and the Lord taketh away, but He
is no longer the only one to do so.
~Aldo Leopold

The dawn of history is best seen in retrospect. What some people are confident is a historic fundamental breakthrough can turn out to be just another blind alley. Advertising copywriters thrive on their ability to portray products as revolutionary and novel wonders. What's new sells. For close to a decade some of Silicon Valley's best and brightest invested in a top secret project they believed would change the world — a mechanized mobile platform, sitting half a foot off the ground, that could wheel itself downstairs. Called Project IT, the Segway rolled out in December 2001 as a revolution in interpersonal transport. Sitting atop two large, rubber wheels, the gigantic scooter base includes built-in computers and balancing devices that allow the disabled and the out-of-condition to cover long distances on urban walkways and negotiate curbs and other challenges unimpeded.

The hoped-for revolution in personal transport the Segway was meant to usher in did not occur. At one point a huge factory was ramped up to take thousands of orders and a billion dollars in sales that never materialized. As with much cutting-edge technology — and the Segway does have some ingenious engineering at its heart — what works on the planning board or in the lab does not always turn out so well in real life. The Segway came to look like the creation of brilliant engineers who were not alert to how little people dislike walking. It seems they also neglected to consider the peak flow problem — namely that crowded, bustling city sidewalks could not handle posses of elevated grown-ups on scooters. But after all, many of us simply aren't excited by the prospect of being propelled distances of up to eleven miles at a pace of ten miles an hour on a vehicle that costs as much as a used car. Today Segways are used by Washington, D.C., tourists and security officers whisking around cavernous shopping malls — a market, to be sure, but not the one investors hoped for, given the research and development money they put into the project. Those who ponied up ninety million dollars in the spring of 2000 owned 15 percent of the company. Even before a single machine was built, Segway's paper value was well over half a billion.

Engineers consider them beautiful pieces of engineering. But it is hard not to think of Segways if you watch the animated movie *Wall-E*, which features obese humans incapacitated by their weight who are smoothly and swiftly transported around their cruise liner's decks as they slurp down junk food, hypnotized by ubiquitous video screens.

Motorola 1972

At the beginning it was not at all clear that mobile phones would be any different. Their invention came about mostly as a corporate strategy to keep one firm from monopolizing a set of radio channels that looked as if they might one day be valuable. In 1972, Robert Galvin, CEO of Motorola, learned that AT&T intended to create a truly mobile phone, thereby staking a claim for sole corporate control of all future wireless networks. Galvin understood that if AT&T prevailed, this would not only solidify its control over the cumbersome car phones AT&T was already selling to a limited number of businessmen and the extravagantly wealthy, it would box Motorola completely out of any future broader-based market. In 1947, the Federal Communications Commission (FCC) had put tight limits on the airwaves, so that at any one time only twenty-three different channels could be used for phones in the entire country. The early car phones were extremely expensive and, not surprisingly, rare. In 1948, about five thousand people in one hundred cities could make regular calls — hardly a booming business. A caller had to stop and park his car, wait for up to an hour to get a free line, and be able to tell an operator the whereabouts of the person he wanted to reach. The network was basically a giant shared party line and usually overloaded.

The engineering solution to this congested network had been devised in 1947 but would not actually be put in place until almost forty years later. Richard Frenkiel and Joel Engel of Bell Labs created plans for a system of applied computers and electronics that would carry the signal around a city through invisible, contiguous wireless cells. With such a system covering an entire region, signals could be passed from one cell to another and serve multiple users at the same time rather than depend on access to a few solitary towers.

By 1968, the FCC had dropped its opposition to cell phones and set the stage for the contest declaring that it would sell off the rights to use a certain bandwidth within which a cell system of mobile communication could work. Bell Labs, the engineering heirs of Alexander Graham Bell and the team that had produced the actual plans for the system, was selected to come up with the first operating mobile phone in the United States.

Part of AT&T, Bell Labs had the advantage. Robert Galvin's father, Paul, the founder of Motorola, was already hooked on an AT&T product. The senior Galvin loved driving about with his "mobile" phone in his Chrysler, calling friends simply to show off the fancy gadget. His son Robert did not think that the world needed or would come to want a hulking phone in every car. If Motorola could take those big cumbersome phones and antennas out of cars and homes and make them truly portable, then AT&T would not be granted exclusive control of the airwaves. Shortly after the new year of 1973, the FCC had slated a hearing to consider granting AT&T a monopoly on these airwaves. Robert Galvin was not about to let that happen. He had six weeks.

Motorola was well aware that nearly thirty years before, Bell Labs had invented the first working cell phone using a wireless signal that moved through the air. So they understood that if they didn't show that they had their own device that required public access to these wireless bandwidths, they would lose what could turn out to be a highly profitable opportunity. The race was on.

A memo that a senior executive of Motorola, Martin Cooper, wrote at the end of October 1972 laid it all out. "What the world really needs," he declared, "is a handheld portable phone." He sketched a plan for "a long range project looking at a personal [portable] telephone. We have to do something spectacular."

Some of his colleagues were doubtful. But Cooper's enthusiasm echoed that of President Kennedy from the previous decade. If we could put a man on the moon, then we could certainly figure out how to compress the innards of a car phone into something that could be carried around. The proposal to make a mobile phone was bold, but it was certainly not absurd. Most of the technologies needed to build such a phone — smaller transistors, more powerful batteries, faster-working processors — were already under development at Motorola. Indeed, the name of the firm comes from its first claim to fame, making car radios — a combination of motor and Victrola, the brand name of one of the first primitive hand-cranked record players.

"We had a religion about making personal communications products smaller and lighter," Cooper, years later, told American Heritage Online. This religion rested on a complex and sophisticated set of engineering breakthroughs in the wings that Cooper was quite familiar with.

In the nineteenth century, Jules Verne had imagined that people would be able to talk to one another across long distances. Handheld communicators fascinated science fiction writers and their fans ("Beam me up, Scotty") throughout the twentieth century. In the comics, Dick Tracy depended on the good-guy detective's ability to summon help at the right time by talking into his two-way radio wristwatch. Funding for science and technology surged in the middle decades of what many had begun to call the American century. It had become a matter of national pride that Americans regularly unleashed new technologies in many very different markets. In the fall of 1972, executives like Galvin and Martin Cooper at Motorola believed that the space-age glamour of a working handheld portable phone would wow the FCC commissioners and be just the kind of wondrous product the country wanted.

A working model of an actual portable phone was worth a thousand pages of technical diagrams. At one Motorola demonstration of the new device, Cooper mentioned that the frequency at which these portable phones would operate was 800 megahertz. One of the FCC commissioners had asked, "What's a megahertz?" The officials they had to wow were not electronically literate.

Waves

While one might expect a government regulator of the electronics industry would have a rudimentary grasp of how electricity works, it wasn't the case in the seventies and it has not been an essential criterion since. For most of us electricity is much like air or water. Open a faucet, water flows. Flip a switch, the room lights up. How electrical power is generated, travels around the world, and carries information is something other people take care of.

Electricity travels in waves, like those that arrive on the edges of a pond into which a stone is tossed. Think of a still, round fishing hole on a country farm. As a bass rises to the surface to snap up a mayfly, its motion releases gentle circles that spread outward onto the water surface in regular waves. If we throw a small pebble into the pond's center, concentric, uniform waves will move to its shores from the spot where the pebble lands. If a much larger and heavier stone lands in the center, it makes much higher waves.

The distance from the peak of one wave to the top of the next is commonly referred to as the wavelength. Waves can also be described by how much power they pack. Their absorption depends on the material through which they travel, and their power depends on their amplitude. Frequency is measured in units that are called hertz.

This unit was named after the physicist Heinrich Hertz. Before his death at age thirty-six, in 1894, Hertz was the first to practically demonstrate that electromagnetic waves could be transmitted through free space at the speed of light.

Hertz himself developed a nearly mystical view of the nature of scientific knowledge about electricity and the physics of waves. "One cannot escape the feeling that these mathematical formulas have an independent existence and an intelligence of their own, that they are wiser than we are, wiser even than their discoverers, that we get more out of them than was originally put into them."

A single hertz is one cycle per second — about the pace of a resting athletic heart. Electromagnetic waves that light and heat and power our homes operate at 60 hertz (or Hz). This means that it takes one-sixtieth of a second for each peak to wend its way through the various wires and transformers in which it travels to power our vacuum cleaners, dishwashers, and clothes dryers. Devices that do not require wires operate at frequencies between nine thousand and three hundred billion hertz. *Mega* comes from the Latin term for "million." Thus, one megahertz written as 1 MHz, is a million cycles per second, faster than anyone could count. Wireless cell phones use pulsed frequency waves from 0.05 to over 100,000 MHz. All radio frequency signals are invisible, and they can pass unobserved into anything not encased in metal and deposit energy into anything that contains water, including the human body. Because radio frequency radiation employed by cell phones cannot be seen and cannot be felt by most of us except when strong enough to warm our bodies, it was at first believed to have no impact on living tissue other than heating.

All forms of radiation move in waves. The distance between wave crests provides one way to measure radiation of all kinds. Ionizing radiation produced by X-rays can be tens or hundreds of millions of times smaller than those of radio, television, walkie talkies, pagers, and cell phones. The closer the spacing of waves on the pond, the faster the surface of the water is said to move or oscillate. The smaller a wave's oscillation, the higher its frequency, and the more energy it carries.

The Electromagnetic Spectrum

This chart shows the full spectrum of electromagnetic fields and radiation. The smallest oscillating waves — those of X-rays or cosmic

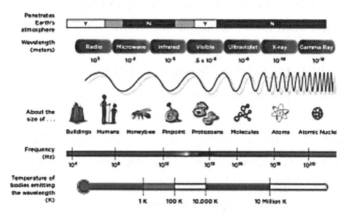

rays from outer space — are in fact most damaging, both in the short run and in the long run. Thus, a single atom bomb blast at Hiroshima and Nagasaki released lethal radiation that killed hundreds of thousands right away and destroyed their homes and neighborhoods. This same solitary blast was shown years later to have caused thousands of others to die of cancer and other degenerative chronic illnesses.

Electromagnetic waves' ability to travel depends on how long they are. The smaller a wave oscillates, the shorter the distance it can reach. Different-frequency electromagnetic waves can be thought of in terms of sounds. A deep, low, sonorous voice projects over a much longer distance, while a high, whiny-pitched yelp does not. If you stand next door, a tinny, shrill chirp cannot be heard, while a big booming bass guitar thunders through the walls. If invisible light rays could be heard, they would be nearly inaudible. Those of X-rays would be completely silent. Cell phone radiation would be louder but still not much more than a whisper.

Of course, Motorola believed that microwaves could and should enable their new phones to work in a completely benign way. All they had to worry about, so they thought, was that the components didn't get hot, or heat up things around them. One of the first medical uses of electricity had been to promote the healing of sore or strained muscles, with a technique that generated an internal warmth and increased blood flow to stressed body parts. Since the healing baths of ancient Rome, it's been understood that the warm temperature can soothe a stiff body. The right amounts of electric current made it possible to heat the body from the inside out. The engineers reasoned that so long as the mobile phones produced no measurable change in temperature, they could not have any other biological effect.

Heat, after all, is nothing but molecules moving faster than they do at cooler temperatures. Heat can be easily measured and easily controlled. With the right insulating materials, or at the lowest level of radiation, heat can become irrelevant.

In the decades following the world's first atomic bomb, the dangers of the most deadly form of energy — ionizing radiation — had become clear to the whole world. Ionizing radiation, such as X-rays and gamma rays, has enough energy, at such ultrahigh frequencies, that it can break the ionic bonds that hold compounds together — throughout the universe, whether that material is found in comets in the solar system or within our bodies. It became a fundamental tenet for some scientists that rays that were not ionizing — like any radiation with longer oscillating wavelengths — had to be harmless. If nonionizing radiation didn't break ionic bonds, and the intensity used was too low to produce any change in temperature, what trouble could it possibly cause?

The first team to create a mobile-phone model simply assumed that it was not possible for radio frequency radiation to have any biological impact. Few at the time realized that low levels of X-rays could cause longer-term health problems, so the lack of interest in the possibility that nonionizing radiation could be a health hazard at that time is understandable.

Alice Stewart was one of the United Kingdom's foremost epidemiologists. In 1998, when she stayed at my home for the evening, we talked into the late hours about the extraordinary challenges she had documenting health risks of low levels of X-rays. She had drawn much criticism in the late 1950s when she began asking women directly to explain their experiences during pregnancy. Until then, medical researchers relied on written records, often difficult to decipher, to determine what patients had undergone during their pregnancies. Having trained as a physician and given birth to two children, Stewart had a keen appreciation of both worlds. Rather than rely on what their doctors reported, Stewart interviewed mothers directly. What she found would change the way the world thought about X-rays. Women who went through X-ray exams during pregnancy had three times a greater chance of producing children who developed leukemia by the time they were age five.

When Stewart first suggested in 1956 that routine exams of pregnant women with X-rays increased the risk that their children would develop childhood cancer, she was pilloried and ridiculed. It was ridiculous, some argued, to think that women would have sound memories of their medical experiences. After all, low doses of X-rays were supposed to be safe. Not until the 1980s, after the medical establishment repeatedly confirmed what Stewart had reported in the 1950s, was the damaging impact of X-rays in pregnancy broadly accepted. Meanwhile, studies continued to emerge from the Hiroshima and Nagasaki atomic bombings, showing that survivors who had incurred lower ionizing exposures to nuclear radiation were developing cancers at much greater rates than anyone had expected.

Given the resistance the medical community had shown to accepting the dangers of X-rays, and the potentially huge markets for products that use wireless nonionizing radiation, the disinterest in exploring potential harm from cell phones is not surprising. Today there is no debate that X-rays directly disturb electrons, break their bonds, disrupt the making of proteins, and impede the ability of cells to fix damage. And yet there has not really been much debate about the potential dangers of radiation from cell phones. It's been assumed they are safe.

This is yet another disconnect surrounding cell phones. The absence of definitive evidence that radio frequency radiation has already damaged millions is a questionable basis for assuming that no such damage could possibly occur in the future.

Our more than ten-billion-year-old universe is jam-packed with naturally generated electromagnetic waves that link planets, molecules, and living matter. Life on earth evolved from the very low-energy Schumann waves that come from the earth's ionospheric resonance to the very high-energy gamma and cosmic rays. Until our societies became electrified with long-wave radio at the dawn of the twentieth century, short-wave radio for warfare in the 1940s, and the more recent growth in microwaves for radar, cooking, and now phones, the level of microwaves in our solar system had not changed for eons. With the advent of our electrified modern life, we and all other living creatures on this planet are flooded in a sea of radiation never before encountered in our evolutionary history.

We live in the age of the microwave. Robert Wilson and Arno Penzias received the Nobel Prize in 1978 for discovering the cosmic microwave and other signals that supported the theory of the big bang that occurred about fifteen billion years ago. This explosive colossus of radiation, matter, and energy gave rise to all the wonders of nature and civilization we observe today. It is sobering to think that the microwaves found in the world today and spewed from that primordial explosion are billions of times less frequent than those emitted by the planet's cell phones and other devices.

The current recommended maximum exposure guidance level for man-made radio frequency radiation that is used worldwide is over a trillion times the natural level that we were exposed to less than a hundred years ago. The last national survey of radio frequency radiation in the United States was conducted three decades ago.

The Race

People who become engineers usually don't get much training in the origins of the universe or human biology and aren't always in great physical shape. But Cooper and the other fellows running Motorola in the early seventies included a few hard-core athletes. Their friendly competition extended to the annual tennis tournament, where Cooper usually held sway. Several of the group had applied to become astronauts, a program that required Marine Corps basic training regimens that culminated in days of no sleep, little food, and extraordinary physical challenges. Ray (Rudy) Krolopp was one of those early runners who could often be found pounding the pavement, inside or out, to stay in shape for his favorite wintertime outdoor activity — skiing. Like many men of their "right stuff" generation, the Motorola engineers loved to compete and if that meant staying up all night for a few days to get something done, they were game.

Krolopp, who would become one of the leaders of the effort to build a mobile phone, had a very important personal goal to meet as well. An avid skier, he wanted to get the project done in time to make a long-planned trip out West with his wife. And he loved the idea of beating AT&T at its own game. Bell Labs, then part of AT&T, had made the first phones to work in police cars and thought it was comfortably ahead of Motorola.

Engineers and architects have a long tradition of creating teams that raced to complete tasks, often working through the night to do so. In nineteenth-century France, at Paris's renowned architecture school École des Beaux-Arts, design contests came to be known as charrettes, for the horse-drawn chariots in which plans were rushed to the judges. Teams of architects would compete to draft plans for bridges or buildings overnight that then had to be transported through the streets of Paris on carts, literally en charrettes. It was not unusual to find experts working on last-minute changes while en route. In much the same gung-ho spirit, Motorola research-and development chief Cooper called in Krolopp on the Monday after Thanksgiving, December 4, 1972, and told him he had six weeks or less to build a small device that could send and receive voice messages without wires and could be held in the hand — a wireless portable phone.

Krolopp had never heard of or imagined such a thing. His first response was, "What the hell is a mobile phone?"

The possibility of mobile phones had already captured the imagination of the entertainment industry. Besides Jules Verne and Dick Tracy, Ian Fleming's spy novels had been turned into razzle-dazzle films featuring the dashing James Bond. Double-0-Seven always managed to get the girl and talked into pens, books, or flashlights to reach the good guys and root out the bad ones. In the 1960s Mel Brooks and Buck Henry wrote a television comedy series, *Get Smart,* featuring Maxwell Smart, a character mixing the dashing Bond with Peter Sellers's bumbling detective, Inspector Clouseau.

One of Smart's standard shticks was to speak into what looked like an ordinary shoe:

Operator: "What number are you calling?"
Smart: "I'm calling Control, Operator. . . ."
Operator: "You have dialed incorrectly. Give me your name and address and your dime will be refunded."
Smart: "Operator, I'm calling from my shoe!"
Operator: "What is the number of your shoe?"
Smart: "It's an unlisted shoe, Operator!"

To use or answer the shoe phone, Agent Smart had to take off his shoe. Dialing 117 converted the shoe into a gun but, of course, left Smart unable to make a fast getaway on foot. Throughout the series, Smart would talk into a variety of ordinary objects that became phones, including a wristwatch, an alarm clock, a handkerchief, a magazine, a garden hose, a car cigarette lighter (the cigarette lighter was hidden in the car phone), a necktie, a belt, a wallet, and a jockstrap, about which Smart asked his boss "to please ring only once." The program included a number of other gadgets that were electronically impossible at the time. There was a bulletproof invisible wall in Smart's apartment that lowered from the ceiling, a candid camera lurking under a full bowl of soup that, with each spoonful, took a picture (with a conspicuous flash) of the person eating the soup, and a powerful miniature laser weapon in the button of a sport jacket (the "laser blazer"). Such was the world of popular culture at the time.

As far as Krolopp was concerned, so long as he could produce a phone that could be truly mobile before his long-planned ski trip, he was up to the challenge, even if it did smack of a television comedy routine or a Hollywood movie.

At the time, the only so-called portable phones in the United States were built into cars and weighed more than a two-year-old child — thirty pounds. In order to get those early car phones to work, a hole had to be drilled in the roof to install the antenna. The only thing portable about these phones was that their working parts took up half of the trunk of a Chevrolet Impala and a third of that of a Cadillac, with a cocktail-table-size package of transistors, wires, tubes, switches, resonators, and filters. While car phones had gotten smaller over time, they still required a forty-pound transceiver mounted in a car's trunk that ran to a handset that was screwed into the front seat of the car.

The first car phones were hardly items of great beauty, but they were status symbols. The car phones themselves cost more than most cars at the time — about four thousand dollars in the United States and close to three thousand in Europe. To work, phones also required a hefty one-hundred-dollar monthly user fee. Not intended for the mass market, these car phones were sold to those who traded in status symbols — people like the founder of Motorola, Paul Galvin.

The effort to put phones into cars for those who were not working for the police or military had actually been started in Sweden, by Televerket, which launched a semiautomatic car phone Mobile System A (MTA) in 1960. Those phones weighed forty kilograms, about the same as a sixth-grade boy. The handset looked like a larger version of the old standard black Bell phone, complete with a ten-digit circular rotary dial. The driver of the car had to stop and dial the number from his console.

Maybe Krolopp was more familiar with the idea of a mobile phone than he later recalled, but what did stick in his head was how exciting a time it was. In just three days, with little sleep and lots of debate, the basic design for what it would take to create a truly mobile phone was produced.

It has been said that engineers are the sort of people who might have become accountants but they did not have quite enough personality. But perhaps no one else understands the joy that comes from building something for the first time from the inside out. Americans had heard the voices of their Apollo astronauts, and seen their images, beamed back to earth using phone technologies that Motorola had devised. Applied engineers were living in a golden age.

In less than two months, the Motorola team had created a working and truly portable phone that was not merely luggable but could actually be carried. At the firm's Holtsville headquarters, Krolopp called Cooper and Galvin and others into a room. Cooper told the assembled senior managers precisely how the project would work, detailing the various components that would be put into operation. When he was done, Krolopp moved to a table in the center of the room that had been covered with a blue cloth. He dramatically yanked it off, unveiling the two-and-a-half-pound heavy-plastic brick — with an affectionate nod to Maxwell Smart — called the shoe phone.

"Eyes opened and jaws dropped, because it was really small," Krolopp remembers. People looked at the shoe-box-size model skeptically. But nobody said a word. Their faces said it all: How could all the workings of a phone that now took up much of a car trunk ever get jammed into such a small container?

Cooper issued a challenge: "Anybody who doesn't believe that this can be done in time, get up and leave."

No one moved.

"With the kind of egos we had, nobody left the room," Cooper recollected.

Krolopp got to make that ski trip.

But the race was only beginning. Bell Labs had assumed the effort to create a mobile phone would be a cakewalk as they had much more experience in the area, having produced police car phones in the 1940s and the basic concept of a cell phone system. Of course, nobody was sharing ideas. They presumed no one could catch up with their in-house technology.

Once everyone had signed off on the proposed model phone at Motorola, they then had to go about actually making it into a viable commercial product that crammed all the intricate wires and parts into something that could be held in the hand and weigh less than a gallon of milk. The first challenge was how to condense what Motorola termed the "supervisory unit," what today would be called the signal processor — the unit that works like an internal traffic cop and controls and coordinates all the rest of the device. In cars, this brain of the phone was the size of a thin book and was jam-packed with wires soldering together the inner workings of transistors, resistors, capacitors — all the stuff needed to send and receive information through a telephone.

They were in luck. Everyone understood that if car phones were ever going to take off, they had to become a lot more compact. At the semiconductor plant in Phoenix, Motorola engineer Al Leitich and his engineering team had spent more than a year trying to pack the car phone's supervisory unit into two simple chips. Don Linder, a native Iowan accustomed to the breakneck pace of most engineering challenges, had led about a dozen design engineers on key parts of the effort to make the system fit within what many thought was an impossibly small space. Like Krolopp and Cooper, Linder was a devoted skier and athlete who had his choice of jobs before coming to Motorola and selected the company because of its well-known commitment to pushing the envelope of innovation. "There weren't many companies in the world designing their own integrated circuits for communications equipment," Linder remembers. "The technology was pretty new. . . . It probably represented six to ten man-years of effort — at least four people for a year and a half or more."

On December 11, a memo Cooper wrote commandeered those smaller chips:

The communications division is currently involved in an extremely important top priority development program, which is expected to have a very significant impact on our future growth. . . . It is imperative for the success of this program that we have working chips [as soon as possible].

So the smaller chips that had been intended to be placed in cars got redirected and quickly made their way into the soon-to-be-unveiled handheld phones. The race with Bell Labs was closing.

Linder got his compressed chips on time. The next step was building a filter that would keep the signals from the transmitter and the receiver from cross-talk or interfering with each other. Car phones had filters as big and heavy as a cinder block. The signal each phone received was only a few microwatts, but the one that gets sent out needed to be several watts — a million times stronger — in order to reach back to the tower, explained Linder.

In order for a cell phone to work, it required chips that were not only smaller than any that had ever been created before, but they also needed the power to send information back out to towers or satellites. A number of those on the Motorola team had previously produced revolutionary and lifesaving wireless engineering breakthroughs during World War II that had helped defeat the Nazis.

3

THE WAR THAT STARTED IT ALL

*Our lives begin to end the day we become
silent about things that matter.*
~Dr. Martin Luther King Jr.

L ike many of those working on the early phones, Motorola's visionary leader, Martin Cooper, got his first experience with wireless in the U.S. Navy, where he had served as a submariner. Those slotted for submarine duty were men with the degree of courage needed to handle being underwater at sea for half a year or more at a time. One in five submariners died during World War II. Their cramped, dangerous quarters provided the first deadly proving grounds for much of wireless communication. Declassified military research reveals that what Allied submariners feared had been true. During the war, the Germans relied on an underwater navigation and range finding system — to keep their submarines in contact in ways that the Allies did not crack for several deadly years. Underwater sound waves would be sent out to find solid objects that they would strike before returning to their origin. The speed with which they returned signaled the distance and depth at which schools of fish or packs of submarines could be found. Radar would come a generation later, relying on the same basic concept out of the water that sonar had used under water — invisible microwave radiation is deflected and returned from the solid metal objects they have struck. The use of radio frequency signals to find solid objects in the air was invented in the crucible of war and arguably determined its outcome.

At the end of 1939, the Germans prepared to invade England. But before doing so, they had to take out British air defense. The Battle of Britain — an unrelenting reign of aerial attacks by the Luftwaffe — was waged during the summer and autumn of 1940. German bombs saturated coastal shipping convoys and centers, aircraft factories and air fields — the infrastructure of the Royal Air Force. Eventually bombing attacks rained down on London and other major urban areas in what became known as the blitz. A quarter million German troops stood ready to invade, as soon as the British air defenses had been laid to waste. In London alone, some ten thousand died during this sustained military campaign. More than a million and a half homes were destroyed.

Under siege and under fire, huddled in damp basements and darkened underground train stations, London's ten million citizens endured extensive, sometimes deadly bombing raids. Luftwaffe aircraft, more than three thousand unmanned and unpredictable V-2 rockets, as well as submarine intrusions along their rocky shoreline, added to the daily terror.

No matter how primitive such devices may appear today, throughout the course of the war, whichever side operated the better form of radio communication prevailed. During World War I, a top secret group of American, British, and French scientists devised an apparatus known by the group's acronym ASDIC, for Anti-Submarine Detection Investigation Committee. At regular intervals, like a never-sleeping hammerhead shark sending out sound waves to find its prey, ASDIC released sound waves that would echo back whenever striking a solid body. The angle of the returning wave and the time it took to come back signaled the location, size, and density of the object. Any suspicious reading was immediately relayed to military command. At distances of two kilometers, ASDIC could find a submarine, a whale, or a school of fish and tell the difference — an achievement that made all the difference in the world.

By World War II, radar would prove a more sophisticated means of achieving the same goal — finding solid objects before they found you. But the Germans had the upper hand at the beginning. Both the Allies and their enemies had invested in developing radar projects. When the war began, the RAF had a primitive coastal radar system in place (which relied on relatively long wavelengths). It provided some protection, but the most threatening instruments of war were not those that would seek out obvious stationary targets like harbors and weapon depots. The greatest danger soared in from the air.

As the toll on England's air force mounted, coming up with some way to protect fighter pilots and ships became an urgent problem. Radar and its antennas have to be made small enough that they could travel (sound familiar?) on, say, a plane.

At the time, the radar signals in common use were generated through large magnetized tubes linked by complex wires and were simply too long to work with shorter and thinner antennas. The first radar systems had wavelengths of close to a foot — some thirty centimeters.

Early radar used the same big and bulky transmitter tubes to send and receive signals as did the first high frequency radio stations. Antennas could be several feet in diameter and in height — far too big for an airplane or a water-based landing vehicle like the PT boat.

Throughout the 1930s and 1940s, the development of a compact magnetized tube to create a small wavelength for radar signals was a top secret project in the United States and the United Kingdom. An airborne antenna had to be less than a meter in diameter so that it could fit inside a plane and pick up operating signals of radar that were about four inches (ten centimeters) in length. To generate shorter wavelengths using conventional radio tubes required a more powerful and more compact magnetron than any that existed in the Allied countries.

A Critical Partnership Across the Atlantic

At the time, all radar, whether on ships or guarding the coasts, rested on huge installations of magnets — called a magnetron — packed into large metal tubes. The magnetron included a matrix that, when heated, released electrons that flowed through the central cylinder. Fortunately for all of us, British engineers soon had figured out how to design what was needed. Working by hand to the precision levels of master machinists, they managed to produce a metallic work of art: an exquisitely thin metal tube that generated a radar signal with a wavelength of ten centimeters and sufficient power to reach long distances.

But there were two huge problems. First of all, they had no idea how to mass-produce the finely honed magnetron, the outer surface of which was coated with a nickel matrix made up of radionuclide metals of barium or strontium oxides. Second, because of the relentless German aerial attacks, even if the British had come up with the right production technology, no factories could be kept safe enough from the bombings, nor was there a reliable supply of some of the basic materials.

Using encrypted radio communications in their Enigma code, the German submarine fleet had sunk hundreds of British vessels. This code relied on a typewriter-like machine to send a unique message that could be read only by another person using the same sort of machine. Once the Allies finally cracked the Enigma codes, they quickly got the upper hand in the Battle of the Atlantic. Realizing that if they suddenly began to intercept all German ships, their discovery would become known, they went after only the largest and most important shipments. But the Allies still did not have any way to find fast-moving and elusive enemy planes in the air before they attacked. The big radar installations rested on the ground, surrounded by huge concrete bunkers and barriers. They needed a mobile radar, one that could easily be used aboard fighter planes, and they needed it desperately.

In his account of the history of radar, *The Invention That Changed the World*, Robert Buderi described the top secret exchanges that took place in 1940 between the then-neutral Americans and their embattled British colleagues. The Welshman Eddie Bowen, one of Britain's top defense scientists, sailed from Liverpool, England, to Halifax, Nova Scotia, escorting a large crate loaded with the top military secrets of Britain. Just after breakfast on the morning of August 29, 1940, Bowen oversaw the transfer of this precious cargo to his train en route to the port of Liverpool, where nightly bombs fell. "Inside lay nothing less than the military secrets of Britain — virtually every single technological item the country could bring to bear on the war. Had some freak accident burst the lock off the chest, the platform would have been awash in blueprints and circuit diagrams for rockets, explosives, superchargers, gyroscopic gunsights, submarine detection devices, self-sealing fuel tanks, even the initial germs of the jet engine and the atomic bomb," Buderi explained.

In its official history the U.S. Office of Research and Development deemed this shipment the most valuable cargo ever to arrive on these shores. From Canada's coast, Bowen was met and conveyed by secret armed escort to the Roosevelt administration's chief science advisor, Dr. Vannevar Bush, in Washington, D.C. Within that box sat the small compact magnetron itself — resembling nothing so much as a large clay pigeon in size. Yet the British-honed magnetron was more powerful than anything Americans had ever devised.

The British invention astonished the Americans, who immediately grasped its stunning import. The big problem was how to produce sufficient numbers of these devices fast and get them to work in airplanes at night. Overruling military efforts to take control of this vital project, Bush turned to talented physicists and engineers at MIT, then working in partnership with Raytheon Corporation, to come up with a way to produce thousands of magnetrons fast.

Conflict of interest scruples become inconsequential during wartime — then as now. Knowing firsthand the skills of those at his old firm, Raytheon, Bush asked them to make the critical components. Like many electrical engineers at the time, the chief of Raytheon during World War II, Percy Spencer, had been completely self-taught. From the age of twelve, he had worked on all manner of things involved in electricity, growing up with the spread of the domestic and industrial use of the technology. Bush had founded Raytheon and went on to direct much of the American war effort at the time as one of the president's most trusted advisors. He knew that the Germans already had better radar and some form of sonar. He also knew, as did all of our military command, that without putting radar onto Allied planes the war would be lost.

In short order Spencer's team provided a brilliant engineering solution that allowed the production of 2,600 magnetrons a day, a feat once thought to have been unattainable. Compact, efficient, fast, mobile radar went from being a theoretical laboratory experiment and military fantasy to being a critical tool for the Allies. Radar-producing technology turned out, like penicillin and antimalarial medicines, pesticides, and rocket design, to be one of the premiere technological advances of the war.

All that mobile radar made a big difference, just as Bush had predicted. The *Reader's Digest* reported in a 1958 profile on Spencer:

> *When his first "maggies" were flown to England, the RAF kill rate quickly shot up and their losses plummeted. When America entered the war in December of 1941, fifteen of Spencer's radar sets — sensitive enough to spot German U-boat periscopes — were installed in U.S. bombers. They proved amazingly effective.*

Sailors working on the first ships to have radar on deck noticed that standing in front of the radar antennas for a few minutes made them rather warm — which could be a good thing on a cold, damp, windy ship. I'm not quite sure how they figured it out, but U.S. and UK war veterans have told me that seamen also determined some other benefits of radar. Young men, often adolescents, who worked on the ships were told that it was not a good idea to stand in front of a radar antenna. Of course, being teenagers they had to find out for themselves what this might do. Some sailors got the idea to roast hot dogs by holding them on long swords directly within the beam. Men getting ready to go ashore after months staring at pinup photos of beckoning starlets discovered another hidden benefit of radar beams. Standing akimbo in front of the radar beam for a few minutes warmed their bodies, especially their private parts. Somehow or other these curious young men determined that the warmth of the radar beam rendered them sterile — a condition they would boast about to women they sought to romance.

Radar, perhaps more fatefully, is credited with having allowed the British to survive the war. Radar was immediately put to work by domestic and military air traffic controllers to track moving objects and weather patterns. But without the stress of the blitz, without the threat of all that Hitler represented, radar might never have been mass-produced so quickly and demonstrated its extraordinary usefulness. Bush and Spencer's work with radar and microwaves had been one of the two top priority research projects of the military during World War II. The other was the Manhattan Project — to build the first atomic bomb.

Back to the Kitchen

Like many engineering breakthroughs, the microwave oven came about quite by accident. One day as he stood directly in front of the beam of a working magnetron in his lab, Spencer discovered that a candy bar in his pocket had melted. Spencer had built some of the first electrified machines and factories in New England. After World War II he held more than two hundred patents and the position of senior vice president of the Raytheon Corporation.

Like all forms of nonionizing radiation, 0.9 to 2.4 GHz — microwaves — cannot be seen. But when microwave radiation is sent through fluid or fat that is within a metal container, the waves move out from their origin and bounce off the solid walls. As the electromagnetic forces are released, microwave-size waves — from a tenth of a centimeter to one hundred centimeters — are just the right wavelengths to cause water to boil. If microwave signals are released into an oven, they carom off the walls and heat up any liquids or electrically conductive tissue they encounter — a discovery that would change the kinds of foods we buy, how we cook, and the basic format of our kitchens.

Curious about what exactly had melted the candy in his own pocket, Spencer next placed kernels of hard corn into the beam of a magnetron tube. To the amusement of his laboratory staff, the corn quickly popped and crackled all over the lab. An uncooked whole egg set under the tube's beam proved without a doubt that heat was being created from the inside out. A skeptical assistant peered at the shaking, quivering egg subject to the tube's beam and got his face splattered just as the cooked egg yolk exploded out of its shell. Spencer was delighted. From this sprang the "Speedie Weenie Project," an attempt to cook hot dogs in a metal box into which radar was beamed.

With his cooking experiments, Spencer knew he had done something far more than amuse lab technicians and surprise his wife. He understood that these invisible small rays could be used to generate heat sufficient to cook anything that contained water or any other polar fluid. Thus was born the microwave oven.

In 1945 Spencer applied for a patent on the first "radar range." In 1947, with the war over, the company built the first microwave oven in the world. A metal container with its own water cooling system, the first microwave stood as tall as a man, weighed more than seven hundred pounds, and cost as much as two cars at the time — some five thousand dollars. The first commercial ovens were big and powerful, operating at a power of 1,600 watts. Use was limited to very large restaurants or institutions. Twenty years later many of the kinks in this gigantic corn popper had been worked out and Amana introduced the first kitchen counter microwave, called a Radarange, at the still pricey tab of five hundred dollars.

Using 1,000 watts of power, the new appliances did not fly off the shelves. People proved a bit skittish about the idea of cooking their food with radar. Maybe Radarange reminded people of a war they wanted to put behind them; maybe it was because the early results were wildly unpredictable for home cooks used to regular ranges and ovens. The early ovens worked by sending wavelengths of 915 MHz — similar to many of today's phones. A cook accustomed to taking an hour to roast a chicken would be left with a rubbery, dried, blackened hockey-puck-like chip after the same period using a Radarange.

By the mid-1970s, the name Radarange had disappeared. In its stead arose the generic term "microwave oven." Micro, after all, means tiny. Waves remind us of the sun and sea, and ovens are warm hearths around which we may remember gathering. A microwave oven sounds like a small, warm, and valuable tool. Indeed it is. How could something very small and wavelike that prepared food possibly be harmful? It was an inspired bit of marketing.

As Litton and other companies entered the production of home-based microwave ovens, two things helped nudge the technology. People, mostly women, became more knowledgeable about how to use the ovens. Television commercials with appealing and attractive women boasting of the oven's time-saving capacity provided mirac-ulous cooking demonstrations. Amana trained young women as sales personnel who went on a major city tour to talk woman-to-woman about the virtues of the microwave oven, a ladylike and practical device. Microwaving bacon proved especially popular, as it generated what most regarded as appetizing smells that would waft through buildings. And in a world where women were beginning to have more choices with what to do with their lives outside of their homes but still were expected to feed their families, anything that meant less time spent in the kitchen while keeping up the obligatory role of homemaker fit easily into the modern home.

Because they did not evenly distribute heat, those early ovens required stopping every two minutes to rotate larger pieces of meat or chicken to ensure that they would cook evenly. Without this stopping and turning, some areas overheated and others remained cold — so-called hot and cold spots. One fellow who worked at Cornell University to improve oven performance remembers how the solution was developed. "The restaurant school complained to us engineers. Trying to heat up dozens of bowls of sauces in the huge oven proved dangerous and impractical because the sauces would get overcooked in some areas and remain cold in others. So we came up with a rotating platform in the base of the oven to ensure more uniform heat."

The solution to this was simple: If microwaves could not directly reach all regions of solid objects evenly, then the solid objects could be made to revolve slowly on plates that soon became standard parts of ovens, or stirrer blades could be used to ensure more uniform distribution of microwave signals throughout the food. Despite concerns raised in part by their own operating manuals, which cautioned of dire consequences from misuse, and warning signs for those with pacemakers in their chests to keep a safe distance away, microwave ovens eventually came to be seen by most as safe and sensible and absolutely essential to the modern kitchen, much like a toaster, refrigerator, or dishwasher.

Microwave oven user guides warn people to be careful about hot fluids — most ovens boil a cup of water within two minutes. Foods heated from the inside can build up pressurized steam. That's why most ovens come with an automatic five-second chime that tells us when it's safe to open the oven and not get splattered by last-minute eruptions of bubbles of heated liquids.

In the beginning, some cell phones relied on wavelengths close to those used by earlier microwave ovens and by primitive radar. The chief difference between phones and ovens is that the power or wattage needed to operate radar or a microwave oven — about 1,000 watts — is much greater than that needed for a digital cell phone. Whether sending voice, photo, or text, cell phones use pulsed peak signals that operate at about one watt and average signals that are a fraction of that. Sending text messages uses less power than speaking. Of course, ovens require one thousand times more power to cook an egg or boil water, but they use the same wavelength as 3G and 4G smart phones — more than two billion cycles a second. It takes just a few minutes to prepare a frozen dinner in a microwave oven. There is growing evidence that effects of microwave radiation add up over time. What happens to our brains after hours and years of using a cell phone that works at less than one watt of power but at the same frequency as an oven? Of course, unlike microwave ovens with their rotating plates, we do not stop and rotate our heads every two minutes to ensure even distribution.

So long as we are not using our cell phones while standing in closed metal boxes — think elevators and trains — microwave exposures from mobile phones are not confined, but free to radiate in all directions. Somehow I do not find that a comforting fact.

From Clunky to All-Powerful

At first, Krolopp wondered what Cooper was talking about. Why bother trying to invent a phone you could walk around with? What was his company getting into? Nobody was going to use these things, Krolopp thought. But it turned out, at least from the perspective of corporate profits, to be a brilliant move.

Cooper knew that AT&T had requested sole control over frequencies between 806 and 881 megahertz. If one firm were granted this dominion, it would effectively shut out all others. Seizing the strategic moment, Motorola allied with General Electric, GTE, RCA, and the Electronic Industries Association to convince the FCC not to give AT&T exclusive control over the airwaves, but to keep the airwaves open for all of the companies — a decision that would come back to haunt many.

However, when Cooper stood on a Manhattan street corner near the Hilton Hotel and placed the first cell phone call — on April 3, 1973 — the person answering was Bell Labs' research chief Joel S. Engel, the fellow who had come up with the idea of cell phone systems in the first place. Competitive engineers were capable of trash talking. We don't know what Engel may have replied, but we can be sure he was not happy. Cooper remembered that people were agog as he strolled down a Manhattan street chattering on his brick-like phone, even daring to cross the street while talking. A decade later the first two-pound phones sold out at close to four thousand dollars apiece — the military prized them and so did a certain kind of affluent geek who didn't mind recharging the battery after less than half an hour.

Why did it take a few days to design a cell phone, but a decade before they were put into widespread use? The initial press release from Motorola in 1973 boasted that phones would be available widely in three years. But phones can't work without a network of towers to support them. It takes time and money to build towers and it used to take time and money to get permission to locate them. But that is no longer the case. The Federal Telecommunications Act of 1996 basically bars local authorities from considering health concerns in deciding where towers can be placed. As to devices themselves, it was easy to convince the What-is-a-megahertz? FCC and its sister agency on cell phone regulation, the FDA, that there was no need to test the safety of these devices. Because cell phones produced no heat, it was assumed that their invisible waves did nothing harmful. That would prove to be one of many wrong assumptions.

Once produced, even at those expensive prices, the first cell phones took off like one of those successful rockets then being launched by NASA, as techno dreams came true. American technology soared again. And all this occurred in a culture that had little understanding of what radio frequency signals were or how they worked.

While some government officials had little grasp of electromagnetic radiation, that was not true of the FDA — at least for a while. The man who for more than a decade shaped FDA directives on cell phones, Mays Swicord, had produced important basic research in his electrical engineering doctoral thesis at the University of Maryland. Swicord showed that radio frequency signals at precisely the same frequency range being proposed for cell phones could disturb the DNA deep within the center of brain cells. He left the FDA in 1994, the year that the agency approved cell phones for general use without any safety testing at all. His role in the matter is unknown. His new job? He became a senior researcher with Motorola.

For years, Swicord was a highly respected researcher who served as editor of the *Bioelectromagnetics Society Newsletter*, a journal that reports original data on biological effects and uses of electromagnetic fields, and also played an influential role in the management of *Bioelectromagnetics*, the main technical journal in the cross-disciplinary fields that drew together specialists in physics, electrical engineering, biology, radiation, and other disciplines that were just then emerging. In 1997, an important paper by Motorola-supported scientist Jerry Phillips appeared in Bioelectromagnetics, showing that genes of rodents exposed to cell-phone-like radiation looked significantly worse than those of unexposed animals. After his study had gone through review and been accepted, the published paper appeared. But it ended with a mysterious final sentence that Phillips did not write, did not agree with, and had refused to include. That added sentence said that the change in gene expression following cell phone irradiation "is probably of no physiologic consequence."

In other words, we have made something happen biologically, but we don't think it is important.

Motorola had helped pay for the study. Phillips reported that during the review process Swicord had asked him to include this sentence and he had refused. When asked about the origins of this qualifying phrase in Phillips's paper, Swicord dismissed Phillips's allegation that he had interfered with the paper as "pure nonsense." By the time his paper appeared with its orphaned final sentence, Phillips no longer worked for Motorola and lost his funding from Defense Department–associated sources as well.

The need for more research in this field is one fact upon which all parties have usually agreed. The absence of research has become part of the rationale for making no changes in the meantime. The history of what little research has been conducted in the United States on radio frequency radiation shows a remarkable pattern of science lost and found repeatedly. Using the Freedom of Information Act to locate the memo, *Microwave News* reported that in 1993, the FDA had concluded that several studies showed that microwave radiation increased cancer risk. But by May 1997, in a letter provided to the U.S. Congress, the agency took quite another tack (echoing a much earlier but not widely known report to the Department of Defense of 1972 referenced online), declaring:

Little is known about the possible health effects of repeated or long-term exposure to low levels of radio frequency radiation (RFR) of the types emitted by wireless communications devices.

And in February 2000, the FDA officially advised that the National Toxicology Program should test radio frequency radiation for its potential to cause cancer, noting:

There is currently insufficient scientific basis for concluding either that wireless communication technologies are safe or that they pose a risk to millions of users. A significant research effort, involving large, well-planned animal experiments, is needed to provide the basis to assess the risk to human health of wireless communications devices.

All of these research questions were raised by the Department of Defense at the time the first mobile phone was created in 1972, by the FDA in 1993, and again in 1997 and 2000, and at the Environmental Health Trust Expert Conference in 2009. But they remain unanswered today — some two decades since cell phones began to be broadly used in America.

And Now, Ladies and Gentlemen, the Smart Phone

Cell phones today contain a number of components, probably the most amazing of which is the circuit board microprocessor, or basic brains of the phone. In the 1950s the U.S. Department of Defense had the best microprocessors in the world, but they were no match for those of today. What once took up hundreds of square feet now fits into the back of your smart phone. Of course, all phones also include a liquid crystal display where images, letters, and numbers can be seen and sometimes pressed, and they also have a built-in microphone, a rechargeable battery, and more and more of them have speakerphones.

These compact devices are small microwave radios. In order to get and give signals, cell phones rely on small amounts of electromagnetic radiation in the form of invisible waves of radio frequency energy that move at the speed of light. Just like the ripples on the pond, the smaller the waves, the less distance they can move and the more power is needed to send them long distances.

Over the past four decades, cell phone types and uses have changed radically. The first bulky, heavy phones relied on analog signals that were basically on all the time without interruption, putting out up to two watts of power. By the late 1980s, an array of such systems ran around the world, including the Advanced Mobile Phone System (AMPS) in North America, Asia Pacific, Russia, Africa, and Israel in the frequency band between 800 and 900 MHz, and the Nordic Mobile Telephone (NMT) 900 system since 1986 in Scandinavia, Netherlands, Switzerland, and Asia.

Radiation from these big old phones was believed to do nothing to living tissue except produce modest amounts of heat.

Modern digital phones provide a compressed way of sending and receiving voice and other information over long distances, using smaller and more powerful signals that are pulsed rather than continuous. The signals from cell phones can be compacted into strings of ones or zeros that the computers understand; that is to say they are digitized.

Digital devices of newer 2G and 3G phones are Formula 1 race cars on the information superhighway, compared to the donkeys Galvin and Cooper envisaged. Launched in the early nineties, these sleek speedster phones use pulsed digital signals powered at up to two watts; 3G and 4G phones use a wider bandwidth usually at much lower power. They continually send digitally pulsed signals to base stations to get new information. As a result, with their off and on signaling 3G phones can result in greater cumulative exposure to radio frequency signals through the usual far-ranging multimedia uses to which they are put day and night.

At the time that the first cell phone was constructed, whatever scientific research had been done on bioelectromagnetics for the most part fell into one of three distinct categories: Some of the work was classified, especially as the Soviet Union was known to have a well-developed program that used microwave technology to create weapons that remain seldom discussed but widely used. Other research into the use of electricity in medicine to restart hearts, repair badly fractured bones, and heal ripped muscles remained within limited circles of medical science. Finally, small amounts of research on the health impacts of cell-phone-like radiation was under way in restricted laboratories and in a few institutions, many of which were outside the United States.

In order to work, each cell phone has to send and receive signals from a base station, connecting with all other cell phones in the area to form a web of information-carrying radio waves. Most people cannot sense these waves at the instant that they occur.

Gro Harlem Brundtland, Norway's former prime minister and the former director general of the WHO, may have appeared eccentric in 2002 when she reported that a nearby operating cell phone could make her ill. In any case, within five months of her having reported her concerns, she was no longer director.

Perhaps this was a coincidence? "Hell, no," said George Carlo, the controversial man who once ran a multi-million-dollar study on cell phone science for the cell phone industry. "Brundtland did not step down incidentally. This was orchestrated by one of her underlings, Mike Repacholi. What happened was Repacholi was asked by the board of directors of the WHO if there could possibly be any validity to Brundtland's concerns. Repacholi told them that Brundtland must have been crazy."

Other off-the-record sources have assured me that Carlo is wrong on this. They say that Brundtland simply finished out her term. There was nothing sinister about the fact that she stopped heading the WHO at precisely the time that the study of a problem with which she was personally afflicted was under way. That was just happenstance.

Carlo is a colorful man who holds a Ph.D., and J.D. To say he inspires strong opinions is an understatement. He led a major joint industry-government study of cell phones that was overseen by the

U.S. government and funded, but also directed in large part, by the industry starting in 1993.

At the time of Brundtland's warning, Carlo was part of the inner sanctum of those working on radio frequency radiation for industry. As the man who led WHO research on cell phones under Brundtland, Repacholi had chaired a number of efforts to review studies on non-ionizing radiation with the International Radiation Protection Association, a nongovernmental United Nations advisory and educational group, many of whose members advise industry. After Brundtland's departure, Repacholi went on to lead several WHO reports on electromagnetic fields, including a review on the biological effects of non-thermal pulsed and amplitude-modulated radio frequency electromagnetic fields and related health risks that was issued by the International Commission on Non-Ionizing Radiation Protection (ICNIRP) — a group Repacholi helped found and still advises today, as its emeritus director.

The ICNIRP is not directly funded by industry, but a project with which half of its members are tied has had substantial financial backing from the Royal Adelaide Hospital of Australia. One would not think at first glance that a hospital might be a conduit for passing along money. But, in fact, the cell phone industry for many years provided several hundred thousand dollars to the hospital, which passed it on to the WHO Electromagnetic Field (WHO EMF) project. Over the years, the WHO EMF project has evaluated cell phone risks and provided other advice to the ICNIRP regarding electromagnetic and cell phone radiation.

With respect to the WHO Electromagnetic Field (WHO EMF) project and the Interphone brain tumor collaboration that former WHO director Brundtland had placed so much hope in, an unusual set of advisors and reviewers is privy to the inner workings of the group, including many of the industries that the project is supposed to be evaluating. Of course, few people think of themselves as biased. Bias is what other people do, those who cannot curb or resist pressures. But those who become scientists think of themselves as somehow invulnerable to influence. Of course, social circumstances affect the facts that we actually do see, where we find them, and with whom and how we choose to share them. It is not so much that people are directly under the thumb of their sponsors, as that they know that if they want to see their work continue, their students supported, and their conferences and papers published, they need to follow the many unwritten rules of the road. It is far easier to keep doing studies aimed at evaluating whether there is a problem and probing the numerous uncertainties of the field than it is to come up with policies to curtail or control potential sources of that problem while studies continue.

Given the complex money trail through which industry funds have indirectly sponsored WHO projects, in his research on this issue, Donald Maisch, of the University of Wollongong, New South Wales, questions whether independent scientific evaluation is possible. "Such a blatant disregard for the fundamental principles of credible science, as well as WHO's mission on protecting world health, speaks of a desperation to bury independent science at all costs, even if that cost is the integrity of WHO."

There is no question that if Brundtland were to speak out about her personal concerns about radio frequency radiation now, she would receive a quite different response. Ironically, the Internet has allowed people who share Brundtland's concerns about the health impacts of radiation from cell phones to find one another, something they could not do when the first phones were produced. How is the world at the dawn of the twenty-first century different from that of the last regarding what is known about cell phones and health? When I first came across reports that people were worried about cell phones, and that some might be especially sensitive to them, I frankly dismissed them myself. After all, I reasoned, cell phones had to be safe. Some of those complaining about health issues had the intense passion about the matter that one tends to dismiss as not credible. If there were really any serious problem, I reasoned, the governments of the world would not blithely underwrite the global spread of this technology. Having spent the past six years learning what some have known for more than four decades, I now understand I was mistaken.

Cell phones have revolutionized the world. We can connect to the mountains of Afghanistan and the centers of collapsed buildings. Cell-phone-like signals fire drone missiles, and find and repair invisible breast tumors. Cell phones provide rural women in South Africa, Nigeria, or Senegal with unprecedented business opportunities to sell, barter, and buy cell-phone-related services, ranging from banking to weather predictions. But is it possible that the pervasive use of cell phones is causing a host of subtle, chronic health problems today, damaging our ability to have healthy children and creating long-term risks to our brains and bodies? The fact that we do not have clear answers to this question at this point in the history of electronic technology is not an accident.

4

WHAT THE ANIMALS TRY TO TELL US

Since the days of revelation, in fact, the same four corrupting errors have been made over and over again ... worst of all, concealment of ignorance by a false show of unheld knowledge, for no better reason than pride.

~Roger Bacon

Of course, it is cruel to take hungry rats and see how much microwave radiation could cause them to stop trying to find food. But many of us think it is far crueler to allow our children to be subjected to such exposures when we aren't sure what this radiation might be doing to them. It is not that some haven't tried to answer these questions. For more than half a century scientists have studied behavior patterns in lab rats and mice in order to predict how certain exposures are likely to affect humans. We study animals not to torture them, but in an effort to predict how humans will respond under the same circumstances.

The word *science* comes from the Latin term scire — "to know." Ideally, modern science works by relying on standard and reproducible scientific methods and technologies to understand the world around us. Of course, science is limited by measurement techniques, but it is even more limited by political and economic circumstances that determine what questions are asked, who gets to answer them, who funds research, and where and when that work becomes public. As results are obtained on any given project, scientists submit their work for review by other scientists; and when and if it passes muster, that work gets published in one of what is still a growing number of scientific journals.

Contrary to the idealized public notion of the whole process, revolutions in scientific thought can be messy, protracted, even deadly. In the seventeenth century, Galileo spent the last years of his life forced to publicly recant his view that the earth moved around the sun and swear his allegiance to ecclesiastical views of the world. Second, scientists themselves, even those with big, bold ideas, can be petty, blustery, backbiting, and vindictive. The discoverer of oxygen and one of the most inventive scientists of his generation, Lavoisier was guillotined in 1794 during the Reign of Terror of the French Revolution. Some claim that Lavoisier lost his life because he had also been a tax collector who had dared to criticize a scientific device invented by a leading revolutionary opponent of the government, Jean-Paul Marat.

For remaining within the accepted conventions of their fields, scientists are rewarded with grants, publications, and invitations to travel the world exchanging information. The impulse to share routine work with other scientists is tempered by the fact that at its core science remains a competitive enterprise. Special rewards are bestowed upon those who appear to have made original contributions. Arguments over who really came up with a given idea first are common, as are retorts to diminish the contribution of others. In 1859, Charles Darwin rushed into print with his ideas of evolution after having learned that Alfred R. Wallace was preparing to submit his twenty-year-long study of the same idea. In the seventeenth century Isaac Newton and

Gottfried Leibniz sparred over which of them should properly be credited with having devised calculus, and their followers continued the dispute for more than a century. James C. Watson, Nobel laureate for his work determining the twisted helical structure of DNA, went to great lengths to minimize the contributions of the young, talented Rosalind Franklin to the enterprise in his memoir of that work. Yet, historians note that the double helix concept would not have been possible without Franklin's brilliant X-ray crystallography images. In Thomas Kuhn's influential analysis of innovations in science, *The Structure of Scientific Revolutions*, published in 1962, the world of science is divided into two major domains: The puzzle-solving work of the majority of scientists involves applying and refining agreed-upon methods and paradigms that are used to characterize the world; others break new boundaries and break out of normal paradigms by devising innovative approaches and new ways of looking at old problems. As science becomes bigger and more expensive, opportunities are reduced for forging new approaches that become recognized as breakthroughs rather than dismissed as deviations or aberrations.

The modern study of how electrical and magnetic impulses affect living systems — what is today called the field of bioelectromagnetics — officially came into existence as a formal discipline less than three decades ago. But the field has roots in scientific discoveries that are more than three hundred years old. In the middle of the eighteenth century, the morbidly curious Italian physician scientist Luigi Galvani wondered why dead frogs' legs would twitch when their bodies were hung up to dry on an iron fence. He deduced that the drying metal produced an electrical current, causing the frog legs to spasm with energy just as a lightning strike does to a metal key on a kite. Within a few years, Galvani was using electrical current to treat fungal infections and tumors. In France, the ingenious researcher Jacques-Arsène d'Arsonval applied a similar logic to the treatment of a host of maladies using high frequency current to warm sore tissues, cauterize leaking blood vessels, and treat various maladies by speeding up blood flow.

Intense disputes over the discoveries of calculus, evolution, and DNA have arisen throughout the past few centuries, but they don't seem to matter much to our ordinary lives. In contrast, controversies that surround efforts to devise, refine, and promote electrical and magnetic technologies that directly and obviously bear on our daily, even hourly, lives remain intense and unresolved. These scientific controversies play out on a field dominated by large investor interests that control the research agenda and release of results. Corporations invested in cell phone technology are rewarded by getting to market first with the newest products. They are not necessarily rewarded for time they might spend developing the safest product.

In fact, as with many other branches of public health research, bioelectromagnetics cannot easily be separated from the economic and political forces that demanded its existence. The Bioelectromagnetic Society (BEMS) officially came into existence as a formal discipline more than three decades ago, in 1978, driven in part by the phenomenal growth of telecommunications, the surge of medical uses of electricity, and by the need for industry to point to a body of research exonerating its products. In a very real sense, BEMS arose as a forum to counter the fears elicited by Paul Brodeur's book about microwave radiation, *The Zapping of America*, an exposé of scientific and political developments surrounding the proliferation of radar and microwaves.

Industry set out to support research as a way of asserting its good intentions. Expectations were straightforward at the time. Since it was firmly believed by those in charge of the business that radio frequency signals could not possibly have a biological impact, supporting these studies was a way to shore up that belief. In 1980, the society created its own journal, *Bioelectromagnetics*, with major support and editorial control from industry as well.

But not all journals, even those formally listed in the National Library of Medicine's PubMed system, are of equal standing and independence. Sometimes journals require that scientists pay to publish in them to underwrite the charges of publication. As you might imagine, this tends to lead to a certain bias, as only those with available resources can afford to pay hundreds or thousands of dollars to print their work. Medical and technology industry firms will underwrite publication as a way to encourage the exchange of information. Often the matter of bias is much more subtle. Conferences are convened by high-sounding nonprofit groups, like the Electric Power Research Institute, that can provide accommodation at, say, posh resorts on California's coast and generous funding for graduate students. The independence of the scientific process is thus subject to pressures and influences that are complex, sometimes subtle, and often impenetrable.

The Science of Cell Phones

With respect to cell phones, the scientific issues at first seem straightforward. Cell signals are weak, invisible, and fast as the speed of light. Radiating out in all directions, at very low power radio frequency, radiation cannot heat human tissue. Some physicists make a simple and attractive case: If radio frequency radiation cannot induce heat, it cannot cause any other problem. It violates the basic laws of physics to think that low-powered cell phone signals could possibly harm living tissue, so we are assured. Yet science tells us that all energy is conserved. If radiated energy is not transformed into heat, then it must have somehow been transformed into potential, kinetic, or chemical energy.

Some of the things that we would like to know about human health cannot be known right away but only after decades have elapsed. In order to predict what will happen to humans, scientists have devised experimental models and methods for studying laboratory animals and cell cultures. People have an understandably morbid fear of cancer or Alzheimer's disease and may not appreciate that by the time these diseases have been diagnosed, they have been brewing a very long time. An invisible cancer cell must double thousands of times before it can be detected, even with powerful technologies such as computerized tomographic scans and magnetic resonance imaging. The latency — or period of time that lapses between first exposure and the development of cancer or Alzheimer's — can be decades.

Medical science is now finally understanding that because the causes of chronic diseases can take decades to be detected, we should not wait for definitive human evidence. If we want to prevent human harm, we have to rely on experimental studies to predict risk rather than using human studies to prove that harm has already happened. In fact, there are a few dozen compounds that we know definitely cause cancer in humans. Most of these human cancer causes are industrial workplace hazards, like asbestos and benzene, or drugs such as those used in hormone replacement therapy, where we have been able to tally cancers in those who endured heavy exposures over long periods of time.

Here's where we have much to learn from animals. Every compound that we are certain causes cancer in humans also produces it in laboratory animals when adequately studied. In the standard test of one hundred laboratory rodents over two years of time, we expose lab animals to different levels of suspect compounds and determine whether they develop more cancers than animals without such exposure. In these studies, each rodent represents about three hundred thousand odd U.S. citizens. At the end of the study, if we have found an increased cancer rate in exposed as compared to unexposed rodents under controlled conditions, then we should assume that the risk will also occur for us.

Rather than wait for body counts to amass for cancer and brain defects in ourselves, scientists today can rely on these and other experimental models to identify avoidable risks. Other shorter-term experimental methods have been developed to predict human risks that do not take years to carry out. Determined to prevent harm, rather than to confirm its occurrence, basic-research scientists have come up with a number of what are called in vitro, or living cell, techniques to try to predict damage from various agents so that we are not forced to wait for the bodies.

The problem that has arisen around cell phones is that the science machine, the system that produces research papers and conferences and dissertations, has become disconnected from the reasons why we study radio frequency radiation. We experiment on animals in order to prevent future human harm, not in order to prove why past damage has already occurred.

The Men Who Saw DNA Ripped Apart

Henry Lai is a soft-spoken, bespectacled man who has spent much of his professional life trying to understand the basic processes that give rise to cancer and other chronic debilitating illnesses. Though diminutive and compact, he is a lot tougher than he looks and has amassed a distinguished record of scientific research, unraveling the nervous system and the ways that our basic genetic material, our DNA, works to repair and prevent damage to our cells from becoming permanent. Within every single one of our trillions of cells, DNA sets the master plan for our bodies. It works like a collection of blueprints that ultimately determine your sex, your movements, your digestion, your brain, and how resilient you are. What makes DNA so remarkable is that every single one of our cells contains a fast-moving mechanics manual that can figure out how to respond to life by tapping the basic ingredients contained within it to keep us alive and well.

Lately Lai has worked on nutritional interventions as a research professor in bioengineering at the University of Washington in Seattle. Lai's group has shown that several specific varieties of Artemisinin — a naturally occurring compound that comes from daisies and is a cousin of tarragon and sagebrush — can arrest the growth of breast cancer cells. Despite his own Chinese heritage, Lai did not start out with a keen interest in herbal medicines. He ended up focusing on Chinese herbal remedies when funding for his first interest — the impact of radio frequency radiation on DNA — dried up.

Every cell of our body contains the basic chemical building blocks that tie together the twisted parallel strands that make up our DNA. Our genetic material consists of a dot that is ten thousand times smaller than the period at the end of this sentence. Within this invisible ball are two strings that, if they could be pulled apart end to end, would be two meters long — as tall as a short basketball player in the NBA. These two threads are held together by an exquisite set of nucleotides that work like connecting ladders made up of hydrogen, nitrogen, phosphorous, and carbon. These ladders can be broken whenever they are damaged; sometimes they can be fixed. What breaks them and what fixes them is the preoccupation of a growing number of experts around the world today.

How DNA is organized determines what genes get turned on or turned off, how proteins are made or absorbed, and ultimately how DNA responds to the usual threats of daily life. DNA works by setting the plans for each living organism, using messengers of RNA to take the basic operating plans and translate them into action.

In 1992, Narenda P. Singh, a researcher whose wife had just started working as a physician at the University of Washington in Seattle, came to Lai's lab with an offer he could hardly refuse. He would work with Lai for no salary on a new method he had invented to examine DNA. Using a simple cooled gelatin-like compound — called agarose — Singh had found that running a weak current under the gel could cause particles within various compounds placed on it to distribute in a predictable pattern. DNA consists of chains of nucleic acids that are linked by sugar-phosphate backbones that naturally have negative charges. When electricity is applied to this for twenty minutes, proteins are arrayed in the gel that are attracted to the positive electrodes and display the structure of normal DNA.

Cells from various body parts can be grown in a test tube or on a plate in a dish and then applied to the gel to depict their central DNA. When these same cells are exposed to a test agent, like sunlight or a toxic chemical, a stain can be painted on them to reveal if this agent affects the structure of their DNA. When examined with a high-powered electron microscope, undamaged DNA has a nice round, compact shape. But if the test agent has disrupted the DNA, then the ball begins to unravel, leaving tiny rivulets or tails much like those of a shooting comet — hence the name "comet assay." Assay simply means a kind of test.

The more tails there are and the brighter they look in the stained results, the greater the score for the damage. Tails can indicate the type of damage and whether there are either single-strand breaks in one piece of DNA or double-strand breaks in both of the parallel helical segments.

Working with Singh, Lai decided to do something different. Rather than exposing cells in a test tube or Petri dish, the investigators used living rats and subjected them to just two hours of radio frequency radiation at about the same level then being used in cell phones. After this exposure ended, brain cells were taken from the animals and evaluated. The results were troubling right away — DNA from the cells of the brains of the radio-frequency radiation-exposed rats was not normal, but broken. The broken brain cells found in these cell-phone-exposed animals are the same as those known to occur in cancer. To remain healthy, DNA needs to remain intact. In the Lai and

Singh study the ties between the double strands of DNA splintered in exposed cells, leaving a long, bright trailing tail. New and dangerous compounds had formed inside the DNA — free radicals now known to give rise to cancer and other serious health problems. It was the first time anyone had seen direct evidence that cell-phone-type radiation adversely affected DNA. It was 1994.

Short-Term Effects

Cancer and Alzheimer's disease scare us, but these long-term illnesses are not the only thing we need to think about with cell phone radiation. We have to ask what prolonged and unprecedented radio-frequency radiation may do to the working of our brains and those of our children. Scientists in Russia, Greece, France, Austria, and Switzerland are producing revolutionary new research on immediate impacts of radio frequency radiation on the brain and our health. Russian scientists have found that repeated radio frequency electrostimulation of one part of the rat brain called the hippocampus results in epilepsy, inducing the brain's neurons to fire out of control, resulting in quivering, spasmodic fits.

How do we figure out whether signals that induce convulsions in animals create problems for us? Of course, it would be unethical to conduct experiments on our children in this country. For the past five years scientists in Moscow have been following two groups of children between the ages of five and twelve — one of which uses mobile phones and the other not. Every year these children are subject to a full battery of psychological and physiological tests. The Russian researchers found changes in the working of the brains of cell phone users ranging from decreased capacity to work, increased fatigue, decrease in attention and semantic memory, and significant loss of the ability to tell the difference between different sounds. Children who are regular cell phone users have a host of what may be called functional problems —

difficulties with learning and behavior. So far, their brains do not look to be different at all in terms of their structure, but the brains of those who are regular cell phone users just don't work as well.

In addition, there are important lessons coming from new animal research in this same area. For a dozen years, scientists in Greece have been producing innovative work exploring how regularly used wireless devices affect the ability of rats to learn and remember what they've learned. In a brilliant and creative effort, Lukas H. Margaritis, a distinguished physiological psychologist at the University of Athens, employs real cordless phones, Wi-Fi systems, and baby monitors and sends signals into the cages where the rats live quite comfortably. In a study of memory and learning, the rats are first placed in a cylindrical water-filled metal container and taught how to swim to a platform to avoid drowning — something they naturally learn pretty easily. After they have mastered this task, Margaritis and his team expose the rats in their comfortable cages to various real-life-like exposures to cell phones, Wi-Fi, and the like for an hour. Then the rodent is put back into the same swimming tank where it previously had found the escape platform. Most of the time, the exposed rodent gets confused and swims around in circles, unable to remember what it had learned just a few hours before. By using regular cell phones and other wireless devices the Greek researchers are mimicking the typical frequencies and they are also employing the simple carrier waveform with pulsed digital signals. The poor exposed rats tend to get lost.

Other work by this innovative group finds that the brains of rats whose mothers are exposed to cell phone radiation during pregnancy have cells that look different from those of unexposed rats. Small amounts of pulsed radio frequency radiation leave rat offspring with what looks like a kind of brain damage.

The Greek team is also studying one of the simplest organisms in the world — C. elegans, a worm with a perfectly symmetrical nervous system that can grow back when the animal is cut in half. Even these lowly worms have trouble after some simple exposures. Usually when they are cut in half, their bodies grow back straight and flat and neat and orderly. Those subject to certain types of radio frequency signals, just like those of the modern cell phone, become snarled and bent.

At Columbia University for more than four decades, Professor Reba Goodman has been working with the even simpler flatworm *Dugesia tigrina*. In hearing her talk about her work, one is struck by the surprising elegance of the species she dissects, as well as her own.

"I adore working with such simple creatures that behave so predictably," she said when we met.

She explained her lifelong fascination with marshaling electric current to heal the body. Her laboratory has identified specific genes that can trigger good and bad development of the nervous system of this worm, effectively creating a logical ground for using electrical fields to promote cellular repair and bone growth. But, she wonders, what can such currents do to a healthy body or to one that is very young or especially ill? Goodman has shown that radio frequency and other electric currents can be used to fix damaged arteries and shattered bone. She worries that no one is examining how growing amounts of such currents today will affect the brains and nervous systems of children.

These studies of simple memory lapses in rats and developmental quirks in worms are perhaps not earthshaking in themselves. But how should we proceed with regard to humans? What about the long-term effects on us? Given how long this research has been going on, what have we found out?

From Two Hours a Day to the Rest of Your Life

The human brain is not easily studied, since it cannot be probed without damage. All brains of all mammals come protected by our bony skulls. There is another form of defense of the brain as well, called the blood-brain barrier. Like many parts of the body, this barrier develops as we mature and does not exist at birth. The idea that the brain has a natural protective layer around it arose when scientists noticed that injecting blue dye into the blood turned the body and tissue of an entire animal blue, but the brain remained pink-gray. They reasoned that whatever kept the brain from turning color had a positive value overall. This so-called barrier is understood to protect the brain from taking in the wrong things, like agents that can dissolve the protective fatty sheaths called myelin that surround our nerves. Myelin also grows as we age and keeps our brain cells working well to identify danger, control impulses, and exercise judgment.

Agents can get into the brain if they have the right affinity for fat, the proper number of paired electrons, or some other kind of atomic passport. Fat-loving materials tend to slip right into the brain. Oil and water don't mix, so watery molecules that repel fat don't make it through, nor do those that are large in size.

Under the wrong circumstances, free radicals can make proteins that weaken the blood-brain barrier and also impair the ability to find, fix, or kill bad cells. When the body is under attack from within, it rallies cellular defenders. So-called heat shock proteins form in order to mend problems by making repairs happen when and where they are needed. If blood pressure is high enough, if reactive compounds are set loose in the bloodstream, then these heat shock proteins can wreak havoc in places where they are not usually found. This barrier stops undesirable materials from entering the brain through the blood.

A team working in Lund, Sweden, in the the Rausing Laboratory for Experimental Neurosurgery and Radiation Physics, has come up with a novel way to study changes in this vital brain defense mechanism. Leif Salford, a sartorially splendid, monocle-wearing neurosurgeon, got into the field of radio frequency radiation looking for a way to push chemotherapy into the cancerous brain. He wondered if radio frequency exposures might enable him to open up the blood-brain barrier so that drugs could be introduced to treat brain cancer.

"I knew that the brain usually resists taking anything into it," he said when we met at a conference on the topic in Washington, D.C. "From where I stood as a neurosurgeon treating cancer, all I wanted to do was to crack into the brain chemically so that we could deliver some of the agents that we knew would kill brain tumors."

James Lin was a senior member of the International Commission on Non-Ionizing Radiation Protection (ICNIRP). He had shown a few years before that microwaves could be used to pass a chemotherapeutic agent across the brain barrier, but Salford independently carried out the same work. Some twenty years before Salford's efforts, Allan H. Frey, working as part of the Office of Naval Research, had first demonstrated that radio frequency radiation relaxed the membrane surrounding the brain. With stunning images, Frey showed that a rodent's brain could take up fluorescent yellow-green coloring if the animal was first subjected to radio frequency radiation. In fact, Salford learned the techniques for studying the blood brain barrier when he had visited Frey's laboratory in Pennsylvania in the 1980s. But Frey himself had been advised to turn to other lines of investigation in the 1970s if he expected to continue to receive major contracts to continue his overall laboratory work.

In his studies in the early 1990s, Salford succeeded in opening up the brain barrier with radio frequency and did enhance delivery of chemicals from the blood into the brain of persons with brain cancer. But this then led him to ask another basic question. If radio frequency exposure causes the brain barrier to relax, how do cell phone exposures to the brain affect healthy, normal people around the world today who are regularly using cell phones?

As a result of this work, the Rausing Laboratory of Sweden has produced some intriguing information about what may be going on inside the heads of these confused, disoriented rodents in the Margaritis laboratory in Greece. For the past two decades, they have examined brain cells from rodents and behavior in whole animals, using mobile phone exposures of two to six hours a day under various conditions. Salford has shown that animals exposed to just two hours of cell phone signals, either the old 2G phones operating at about 900 MHz or the newer and exciting 3G phones at 1,900 MHz, were much less able to complete simple tasks at which they usually excelled. Even two months later, exposed boy rats remained just a bit less smart than exposed girl rats. They showed "significant deficits in learning." Just like the rats in Greece — exposure to cell phone radiation renders these animals unable to remember where to go in a maze that they successfully navigated just a few hours earlier.

Examining the DNA and genes of the brain cell of these disoriented rats, Salford's team found that all is not well. Using computers to characterize gene patterns, they show that rats subject to cell phone radiation have more direct brain damage, less ability to fix this, and greater chances of growing and acting strangely. Once the blood-brain barrier is breached, then anything circulating into our bodies at the time, alcohol, drugs, toxic chemicals, cigarette smoke, diesel exhaust, will more readily enter the brain from the blood.

Salford is passing the baton for much of the basic research in this field to Henrietta Nittby, a brilliant young physician who was top in her class in physics. Nittby also holds a Ph.D. for a series of important papers detailing molecular and genetic changes in rodent brains after exposure to pulsed cell phone signals. Using specially designed cages in which animals rest while they receive cell phone signals, she has shown that rats exposed to cell phone signals for just two hours a day for a single week begin to leak microscopic fluid from their brains into their blood. When it is healthy, the brain of rats and humans is full of fat and is well insulated to keep out anything that is watery. Careful analysis of the brains of the cell-phone-exposed rats shows that after just a week of regular two-hour daily exposure they release albumin — a critical material that should not be found escaping from the brain. As a result, these rats remain vulnerable to taking in other agents in the blood that normally would never enter their brains.

Nittby's work also finds that the genes that rodents and we ourselves use to repair the regular attacks of daily life are severely impaired after just two hours a day (for one week) of cell phone exposure. In other studies of animals that have been exposed to cell phone radiation for close to a year, Nittby finds that their brains look perfectly normal under the microscope. But while the structure of the brain looks normal, the way the brain works is not normal at all. In effect, these rats show evidence of forgetfulness, senility, and loss of memory.

The Lund team concludes one of their most recent publications with an unusual warning. They note that, of course, the intense use of cell phones by children is unlikely to induce any obvious, dramatic, or immediate impacts on health. "It may, however, in the long run, result in reduced brain reserve capacity that might be unveiled by other later neuronal disease or even the wear and tear of aging. We cannot exclude that after some decades of (often) daily use, a whole generation of users may suffer negative effects maybe already in their middle age."

Science proceeds in its one-step-forward-two-steps-back awkward way. A dogma exists, and then gradually more and more findings come in from the edges of the scientific world that suggest the dogma must be overturned. Yet there is no denying that the majority of published studies on radio frequency radiation and the brain do not show any impact. How is this possible? Frey reflects back on the research enterprise some four decades later with a bit of cynicism. "Those who set up studies that are supposed to replicate work on the blood-brain barrier, can make changes in the design that are small but critical. Basically what is supposed to be an identical experiment with contrary results turns out to be no such thing. Instead, studies are done not to clarify the problem, but to confuse people. We've got quite a history of that in this field."

In fact the ability of radio frequency radiation to weaken the blood-brain barrier was first demonstrated nearly four decades ago. Most of the studies that find no problem have been sponsored directly by the industry and have used slightly different approaches. The generation of negative studies in this area, as in many topics relating to the cell phone science, has been deliberate and effective until now. A tipping point arrives when the way things have appeared to work no longer makes sense. I believe that in the scientific world, we have arrived at that tipping point.

5

AN ELECTRICAL STORM IN THE BRAIN

There is more religion in men's science than there is science in their religion.

~Henry David Thoreau

Lloyd Morgan went to lunch at Ajanta, his favorite Indian restaurant, with his buddy Ken Johnson. It was a Friday in early spring, April 28, 1995. As they ate, Morgan spoke animatedly. For months he had been talking with machine-gun rapidity and a bit more excitement than usual. Suddenly, he stopped midsentence. Perhaps for a few seconds, maybe less, he was surrounded by white light, an unbearable aura of uncommonly transforming brightness. A sense of impending doom and dread hit, as though the universe was about to collapse. His life would never be the same. His brain went into a kind of tonic spastic shock and froze. He has no memory of what happened next. No recollection of what happened can ever enter his consciousness. That's probably a good thing.

During a grand mal seizure such as Morgan went through, the entire brain is wracked by a series of unstoppable electrical storms. Internal lightning disrupts the normal wiring of the nervous system.

The vocal cords clamp down on whatever air is in the voice box, producing a primal grunting scream. Unseeing eyes roll back under the eyelids. Unhearing ears become like breakwaters to powerful waves crashing across the entire brain. Sometimes the tongue thrashes about and limbs flail wildly.

The head jerks back, crashing into whatever it hits. Nothing moves deliberately and everything moves at once.

Morgan woke up from this attack in the ambulance. He was one of the lucky ones. He retained the ability to speak, hear, move, and think. In the emergency room at Alexian Brothers Hospital in San Jose, California, he was able to listen to the report of the CT scan.

"You have a massive brain tumor."

He watched the physician point to the films of the intruding growth.

"See these invasive fingers?"

When his luncheon companion arrived at the emergency room, Morgan resumed their conversation without missing a beat. About five feet eight inches tall on a good day and of lean build, Morgan is an unusual man in a number of ways. He talks a lot and his brain is big enough that no one would ever imagine he had lost a significant piece of it to a half day of surgery fifteen years ago. But Morgan is a man with lots to say who knows he may not have much time to say it. Even though his tumor was technically termed benign, the meningioma that nearly killed him is notorious for returning, perhaps somewhere else within the head. Brains don't have much room for things to grow within them.

In the meantime, Morgan was and is a man in a hurry. The seizure gave him a new career — that of brain tumor activist. He spent eight days in "critical condition" waiting for his brain swelling to subside enough for him to go through surgery to remove the tumor. His neurosurgeon, Dr. James Saadi, explained that if they had tried to operate immediately, Morgan's brain might have ended up all over the operating room, because the swelling was so extensive. It's a very good thing for Morgan that he also had a rather large, thick Irish skull, or else he would have died from herniation of the swollen brain inside. When the pressure from a tumor gets too high, the spongy mass gets shoved down into the opening at the top of the brain stem, cutting off the spinal cord, paralyzing the body and ending life.

Right after waking up from brain surgery, Morgan asked the one question everyone asks: "How did I get this thing?"

His physician had read a bit more than most and had an answer — an answer that would change the rest of Morgan's life and the lives of many others.

Dr. Saadi replied that he was not certain, "but, perhaps, electromagnetic fields."

It was 1995 and Morgan was stunned. He had always been one of the smartest guys in the room throughout his schooling and work in electrical engineering. He had been the guy they called in when nobody else could figure out why what had worked well in the laboratory didn't work at all in the factory. A troubleshooter in what was called process engineering for major firms for years, Morgan had worked surrounded by some of the latest electronic production technologies, which he had tweaked and sometimes redesigned. Morgan could figure out why a mistake that happened only once every billion cycles could cause a computer system to crash, and he knew how to fix it. He was well read and curious, like most adults who grow up — as much as they ever can grow up — living in Berkeley. Yet he had never heard that working with electronics could put him at risk of anything other than a certain nerdiness that goes with the field itself.

Having spent his life designing things, Morgan turned his skills toward figuring out what had happened to his brain. He found a trove of information that was sponsored by expert groups. As an engineer, he eagerly read and understood papers from the Electric Power Research

Institute, and other studies conducted for electrical utilities. He was shocked to find out that workers regularly exposed to electromagnetic fields like those with which he typically worked had higher risks of developing leukemia and brain tumors and even breast cancer in men.

In fact, Morgan's rather large, sturdy, and smart head probably saved his life. Because his skull could accommodate the tumor that evolved, he did not develop a stroke or die from the experience. While we cannot be certain exactly what did cause Morgan's tumor, we do know that in his case it had nothing to do with radiation from cell phones. He has never used one and never will. But he did work with electromagnetic fields throughout his adult life. And on this matter, the World Health Organization and many other authorities are clear. Men and women who have close contact with high-voltage switching stations and build and repair electromagnetic equipment that provides the rest of us with the ability to use our toasters and cooktop stoves develop triple the amount of some tumors compared with the rest of us without such exposures.

Within days of coming out of the surgery, Morgan turned his attention to understanding the causes of brain tumors.

He wanted to know about his own meningioma. While meningioma is typically labeled benign, this tumor can in fact be just as lethal as one that is called malignant. He also wondered why so many more young people were developing brain tumors, both malignant and so-called benign ones.

The evidence is clear that our brains are exquisitely sensitive to various radio frequency exposures. In fact, one of the most promising ways of treating brain tumors today involves zapping them with various forms of radiation to destroy cancer cells inside the brain. Our bodies are not one single uniform density but contain many different layers and types of biological tissue, including dense bone, rubbery fat, sinewy muscle, and spongy brain matter. The amount of radio frequency that any biological tissue can take in depends on four things: how often the waves are being transmitted, the size of their tallest waves, the power with which they are being created, and the amount of fluid or fat that makes up the specific tissue. The brains of children have a pretty high fluid content compared to those of adults. This is why shaking young children is so dangerous — literally their brain matter can be sloshed around. Children's skulls and bone marrow are thinner and much more absorptive than those of adults — a fact that explains why children's heads can absorb double or more the radio frequency energy of adults' heads.

Because Morgan's brain was mature, it contained much less fluid and the tumor had less room to grow. Because he was lean, the layer of fat just below the skin of the brain, called the subcutaneous layer, was not as thick as that of a heavier or taller man.

Not many people appreciate that standard limits for cell phone radiation today are based on a man who does not resemble the typical user today. In coming up with ways to estimate exposures from cell phones, scientists in 1996 relied on a fellow named SAM — which stands for Standard Anthropomorphic Man. SAM is not an ordinary guy. He ranked in size and mass at the top 10 percent of all military recruits in 1989, weighing more than two hundred pounds, with an eleven-pound head, and standing about six feet two inches tall. SAM was not especially talkative, as he was assumed to use a cell phone for no more than six minutes at a time. In 1996, fewer than 5 percent of all of us — some fifteen million Americans — had cell phones.

In fact, safety standards for radio frequency radiation in the United States date back to 1962, long before cell phones moved from theory to reality. Many of these standards were devised and revised based on research carried out at the University of Utah under contract to industry for more than a quarter of a century. When these standards were first created, the basic question on everyone's mind was what level of current could kill or shock someone using a particular piece of equipment. The American National Standards Institute (ANSI) set standards for all sorts of electronic devices that were revised every decade, based on the simple consideration of how much current might disturb, stun, or kill someone. But that approach to setting standards would change because of the award-winning work completed in Utah by a team of electrical engineers who started out doing routine, puzzle-solving investigations and ended up devising new paradigms of the way science thinks about the human impact of radio frequency and other electromagnetic radiation.

Cell phones are basically a somewhat complicated radio that receives and sends millions of pulsed microwave-size signals. Within the phone, a transmitter turns the sound of your voice into invisible microwaves of nonionizing radiation that are sent away from the antenna at the speed of light. Standards were originally set for the first generation of analog cell phones (now called 1G), which were always on, in order to prevent overheating of tissue in SAM's head. Unlike the rest of us, SAM's brain was uniform throughout. SAM testing involves pouring a liquid — of varying density for differing MHz — into an empty plastic head about the size of a ten-pin bowling ball. A programmed computer automatically sends an instrumental probe into this liquid to record how much radio frequency radiation reaches specific parts of the skull as a cell phone is held ten millimeters — about a third of an inch — from the ear. Our heads and those of our children, of course, are not one simple, consistent, gooey liquid but contain many different components, including the hypothalamus, amygdala, and bone marrow. But SAM is a simpler fellow from simpler days when the idea that toddlers could be using cell phones was unimaginable.

These standards were set in 1993 and based on SAM's big brain, not for the much smaller heads of children, of women, or other adults.

The SAM-based standards also do not take into account the fact that radio frequency signals have other biological impacts and can increase the pace at which any agent can get into the brain, causing some unusual proteins to form in the blood, which are absorbed much more deeply into the brain of a young child. Nor do any of these models consider that the brain of a young child triples in size in the first year of life and continues to develop throughout adolescence.

A Resonant Researcher

Sometimes revolutions are begun by improbable leaders. Om P. Gandhi and his group at the University of Utah were supported by the Defense Department and industry for three decades as they painstakingly devised the methods that would be used to evaluate the impact of microwaves on living systems. His team started out studying lab rats that had been deprived of food so that they would be eager to learn to perform in a maze in reward for pellets. They soon found that certain wavelengths and conditions of microwave energy could cause these starved rats to stop working for chow. That was how the first standards for exposure to microwaves for the rest of us were set.

For these efforts in estimating maximum safe exposures to electromagnetic power, Gandhi received numerous awards. A seminal paper of 1975 showed that microwave resonance in the human body is between eight to ten times higher than previously believed.

While we may not be aware of it much of the time, our body is always vibrating with the world around us. Because we are mostly water, we rarely sense our own resonance or vibrations. At rock concerts our bodies feel the thundering pulse of the bass beat blaring out through what always seem to me to be too-loud speakers that surround the concert halls or stadiums in which such concerts typically play. But, every day and everywhere, our bodies are silently vibrating at certain speeds called resonances.

One of the most dramatic illustrations of resonance comes from ancient China, where the strange objects known as spouting bowls were made 2,500 years ago. Crafted of finely tuned bronze, the bowls are so precisely produced that when the right amount of water is placed in them and the handles are rubbed correctly, vibrations are generated that give rise to waterspouts. The historian of science Joseph Needham reported seeing spouts as high as three feet. Waterspouts arise because two competing, equal, and precisely opposite waves are generated simultaneously as a result of the vibrations of the bowl itself. The waves start from opposing sections of the bowl and move, at the same speed and height, to come together, like two hands beginning to pray, creating a standing wave. First the water in the bowls ripples, then it begins to vibrate. The bowls start to sing, producing a deep resonant tone that becomes stronger as water stands higher and higher.

By any measure a standing wave is extraordinary. It precisely balances the dispersive forces that normally would destroy it with other, peculiar counteracting forces. The combined effect of exquisitely balanced opposition gives the wave the continued cohesion to prolong its existence.

When we are exposed to radio frequency radiation, again because we are mostly water, most of us are completely unaware of the fact that these invisible signals vibrate with our cells, which have their own natural rate of vibration or resonance. Every physical object has its own resonant frequency, rates at which it will vibrate with the world around it. Things like us that are squishy liquid tend to be of lower resonance and have what is called a low Q factor, while solid metal objects like a tuning fork, a xylophone, or copper wire found in many electronic devices, have much higher resonances and Q factors.

Based on Gandhi's path-breaking work confirming the natural resonance of our bodies and those of animals, ANSI and all the other groups then involved in standard setting revised the safety guidelines, whether for cell phones, electronic surveillance devices, or medical equipment, downward by a factor of ten at some frequencies. Within the decade most national authorities had adopted these changes.

Gandhi explains that by the mid-1980s, ANSI had become a bit antsy about all the public attention being paid to its standard-setting activities. Guys in expensive suits began to show up at meetings, inquiring about what the various scientists were thinking about. People engaged in the effort became a bit wary of where this would all lead. Gandhi explained that "some of these ANSI guys wanted nothing to do with the regulatory world. Their leaders understood that someday someone would file a lawsuit arguing that the standards had not been sufficiently tough. As more and more uses of radio frequency radiation were starting to come on line, ANSI decided to get out of the effort of recommending health and safety standards altogether."

Another group, the Institute for Electronics and Electrical Engineering, now simply called by its initials IEEE, eagerly offered to serve as a forum that would take over the activity. IEEE had been around for more than a century, as a predecessor group of engineers organized around the first telegraphs and early power plants. By the early 1980s, the group remained chiefly an American organization, with more than half of its members coming from industry directly and others drawn from academic engineering faculty.

In the beginning, the IEEE standards simply followed those of ANSI. But the old ANSI C 95.1 Safety Standard was modified in 1992 and reissued as the IEEE 95.1 RF Safety Standard. The importance of this was straightforward. Based on Gandhi's analyses, the 1992 standards for general public exposures became five times lower than those of a decade earlier, for the widely used frequencies of 30 KHz to 300 GHz.

Because of work completed in Utah, it became clear that people can absorb more energy than was previously thought from sources at a distance. Keep in mind that at this time, there were almost no cell phones in use, excepting the clunker shoe and car phones of the business and military worlds.

Something rather curious happened next in the standard-setting world. From 1988, when cell phones started to become commercially viable, until 1996, shortly after the first lawsuit claiming that cell phones could cause brain cancer was filed, Gandhi served as co-chair of the powerful and influential subcommittee of the IEEE that recommended electromagnetic safety standards for all wireless devices. Members of the committee consisted of academic researchers, with some industry representatives. Cell phones remained a fairly rare commodity at the time. All those who led the standard-setting group had been academics. The year that Gandhi stepped down as chair, he also produced a paper that would rattle the industry. The old models had basically used a large, empty plastic bowling ball into which a uniform liquid of specific density had been poured. His new work took into account the fact that our brains are not homogeneous and used anatomically scaled models of the organs contained within the skulls of a young child, a ten-year-old, and an adult male. This work made it clear that our heads are not empty shells and that radio frequency signals were absorbed much more deeply into the brains of children than those of adults.

He then went on to show that heads of smaller adults — actually most of us — would also absorb more radiation than SAM. Up until this work was published, Gandhi and his group had devised the models for how to evaluate cell phone radiation and worked closely and directly with many in the industry producing the new phones. He was called on and testified for the industry in lawsuits about exposures to the phones.

In 1993, when fewer than 1 percent of all Americans used cell phones, the mobile phone industry faced a serious challenge to its public reputation. H. David Reynard filed a lawsuit against the phone manufacturer Motorola; the communications provider NEC; and the store where he purchased the phone two years earlier, claiming that regular cell phone use had caused or accelerated the growth of his wife Susan's deadly brain tumor. The filing of a lawsuit alleging that any technology produces a serious health problem is not easily undertaken. Such a suit only happens after attorneys and experts have concluded that there is merit to the matter and that they are willing to put up the time and money to pay for it. Other claims soon followed. Phone stocks lost more than 10 percent of their value within a week following widower Reynard's appearance on *Larry King Live* discussing the case.

While none of these lawsuits succeeded, they raised public concerns. What does industry do when an issue like this surfaces? They assume there is no merit to the allegations and summon forces to kill the discussion. They tap the best and the brightest to study the problem and keep on studying the problem. Interesting work gets done. Doctoral dissertations and laboratories are well funded. Decades later research is still under way. No one can be opposed to research, after all. Certainly those whose livelihoods depend on it have a strong interest in having questions drawn out. So long as bona fide technical questions remain unresolved, research programs continue to be funded and industry profits are not disrupted.

Paul Staiano, president of Motorola, assured ABC's *20/20* that the claim was completely unfounded. "Forty years of research and more than ten thousand studies have proved that cellular telephones are safe." The irony of this claim was that at the time what little research had been made public on the topic indicated that the microwave-like signals then released by cell phones did have biological impacts.

Staiano went on to claim that radio frequency signals had been with us since the dawn of the world. This is a true statement. But, what he did not say, and may not have appreciated, is that the levels of radio frequency signals that started the only world we know were billions of times less than those that are getting into our heads today around the world. In fact, it is unlikely that Susan Reynard's brain tumor was caused solely by her cell phone use, since she had used her phone for just two years. But it is entirely possible that repeated exposures to the phone may have accelerated the growth of a tumor in her head that had been started earlier.

In the case of Susan Reynard, Gandhi worked as an expert for the cell phone industry and devised a model of the phone she had used. He explained that the position of the antenna on her phone kept it far from the head, thus reducing direct radiation exposure to her brain. In 1995, Gandhi received the highest accolade of his profession of bioelectro-magnetics — the d'Arsonval Medal of the Bioelectromagnetics Society for pioneering contributions to the field. The paper he issued the very next year, showing the much greater absorption of radio frequency radi-ation into the heads of children, basically ended his long and successful ties with the defense and the electronics industries.

Change the Rules?

Based on the new work he had produced, Gandhi called for a revision of the safety standards that regulated cell phones. The indus-try was stunned. For years, Gandhi had been one of those on whom they had counted. If Gandhi's work went uncontested, it would mean that children, women, and men with smaller heads could not safely use some electronic devices or that these devices would have to be redesigned to emit less radio frequency radiation.

The industry's first response was to cut off all of Gandhi's funding. Then they hired other modelers to find flaws in the work. Since Gandhi had trained many of those in the profession and worked closely with industry experts for decades, it was not easy to find anyone to challenge his work. Of course, as is the nature of science in such matters, Gandhi himself would go on to refine this work in later iterations, but the basic findings were not substantially altered. Children's heads were not simply smaller versions of adults' heads — something every parent knows.

The SAM model had not only used a big-guy brain and body as the basis for all standards for everyone, it had assumed that the entire brain was uniform in consistency. While various efforts, including work from Gandhi himself, have advanced the approach, none have altered the basic conclusion: Children's brains are different from those of adults. They are, of course, smaller, but they also are developing at a faster rate. Anyone can understand that when something moves faster, the chance for mistakes to be made is greater. That's why we have speed limits. Speed kills and does so logarithmically — that is to say that the chances of dying while driving a car at sixty miles an hour is a hundred times less than while driving a car at seventy miles an hour. Other models have followed Gandhi's work. Some have offered enhancements. All are agreed — children's brains and skulls absorb at least twice as much radio frequency radiation as those of adults. Bone marrow can take in ten times more radiation in children than in adults, according to reports from Swiss scientists in 2010.

These advances in our understanding of the young brain have not had any impact on the way that cell phones are tested or rated. Yet. The testing lab that runs the SAM models for all U.S. and many foreign phones still basically pours milk jug containers of liquid of various densities into a large plastic head about the size of a ten-pin bowling ball and then tests how deeply into that uniform liquid various signals will reach. Of course, the brain is not one simple entity but a complex of parts. Weighing about three pounds in the adult, the brain itself is shielded by protective coverings called meninges. This is where Lloyd Morgan's tumor began.

So far, the models of the brain used to estimate exposure to cell phones around the world today do not incorporate a number of basic details of neuroanatomy. Alvaro de Salles is an electrical engineer in Porto Alegre, Brazil, near the bottom of the world, who chairs a department of electrical engineering. Niels Kuster is a brain and body modeler from Switzerland who runs a major international institute devoted to radio frequency modeling. While they do not work together, in a series of papers and reports produced over the past decade, they have each been making the case for applying more detailed and biologically based models to the estimation of exposures to the brains and bodies of all of us. De Salles works with a series of brain models that rely on magnetic resonance imaging made from a live ten-year-old boy and clearly shows the different absorption characteristics of different parts of the brain. In Switzerland, Kuster and his team of dozens of experts have come up with models of absorption into the heads and bodies of an entire family ranging from a three-year-old toddler to a young boy and girl, and their parents, including a pregnant woman. While there are disputes about the details, they are agreed: You can dress children to look like grown-ups, but you can't make their brains work like those of adults.

All of these models understand that, contrary to the assumptions behind using SAM to set standards for everyone, when it comes to our heads and brains, one size does not fit all. Thus the ear receives the most radiation. But the acoustic or hearing nerve also gets a fairly high dose, as does the eye and the area right under the cheek called the salivary or parotid gland. These happen to be areas of the brain and head where some investigators have found increased risks for heavy cell phone users. Could heavy cell phone use explain why Diane von Furstenberg or Roger Ebert developed cancerous tissue under their cheeks? Perhaps the fact that Israelis were the world's heaviest cell phone users in the year 2000 explains why the rate of these cancers has tripled in that nation in persons under the age of twenty?

By 2004, the proposed model for estimating cell phone exposure that IEEE would rely on was altered in a way that Gandhi had never predicted or suggested. The science had not changed but the scientists had. Until 1999, Gandhi had headed up the standard-setting committee of the IEEE and also had devised the models used to estimate absorption into the brain. But a few years later the phones were different and so were those who set the standards for them. The man who replaced Gandhi was C. K. Chou, then a respected electronics engineer with the City of Hope, a major cancer research center. Within a few years, Chou had a new job, heading up Motorola's program of research on radio frequency signals.

In the 1970s, Gandhi had started out studying himself and his students in order to determine how living things are affected by various forms of electrical and magnetic fields, from high-voltage power lines to microwaves and radio signals. How can we determine what radio waves do to the body? Early research in the 1970s put hungry rodents inside microwave exposure chambers to study how low radiation levels changed their food-seeking behavior and to measure how hot they became under various conditions and when they would basically stop working for food altogether.

Gandhi helped craft an entirely new field of research, combining information from basic electrical engineering with that of human biology, creating the field of bioelectromagnetics. This is not a subject for those who are intimidated by calculus or mathematical modeling. For the past forty years, Gandhi has refined these studies as a professor and chair of electrical engineering at the University of Utah. To get a better appreciation of radio frequency properties, he developed a model of the human head. Working with medical experts and using magnetic resonance imaging studies and probes, Gandhi has determined precisely where and how invisible radio frequency signals are absorbed into the head. His work basically laid the foundation for the development of standards to protect humans around the world.

In testifying before Senators Tom Harkin and Arlen Specter on this matter in September 2009, I brought along a sample head adapted from Gandhi's work. A simple pink plastic model of the brain was split in two, one side showing radio frequency absorption from cell phones going about two inches into the brain of an adult, the other showing that such absorption reaches much deeper through the brain of a five-year-old. My colleague Ronald Herberman, then the prize-winning director of the University of Pittsburgh Cancer Institute, had made a similar presentation to a congressional hearing the year before. At the end of Herberman's testimony, Chairman Dennis Kucinich held up the head, like Hamlet remembering the goodwill of poor Yorick. The ranking Republican leader, Representative Darrell Issa, and his colleague Dan Burton as well as Democrat Diane Watson, passed around the brain model, marveling at the depth to which such signals can reach.

I am especially grateful that Gandhi and I have been able to work with de Salles, to produce an important new evaluation of the problem. In a measured but critical tone, when we met to review our evaluation, Gandhi explained that something has gone very wrong with standard setting in the United States in the past few years:

"Starting in the late 1980s, I chaired the committee that set standards for radio-frequency exposures before cell phones ever existed. About a decade ago, C. K. Chou, then at the City of Hope Hospital, replaced me. Within two years, Chou had moved. He became a senior executive with Motorola — a clear conflict of interest. The committee that advises as to cell phone standards is supposed to be independent and had never before been led by someone from the very industry it advises. Under Chou's leadership, the committee relaxed the standards for cell phones as of 2005. Having spent my entire life developing models of the brain,

I know how things work. I also know that what we have done here is to ratchet up exposures, without actually telling people we have done so. Today's standards for cell phones have more than doubled the amount of radio-frequency radiation allowed into the brain."

Why does the change in assumptions used in this model matter? In a series of peer-reviewed papers, Gandhi explained that the new models for industry safety testing do not hold the phone next to the head, where most of us place it. Instead these models assume that the phone is at least a half an inch from the brain. Gandhi believes that for every single millimeter of distance that a phone is held away from the head, the estimated exposure inside the brain is lowered by 15 percent. He also feels that altering the models so that they use the word pinna to depict the plastic spacer, rather than ear, achieves an interesting result. "Nobody knows what you are talking about. *Pinna* might as well be the top of a mountain to most people." He said further:

In the early days of the cell phone, the antennas were external, sticking out almost a foot from the bulky plastic box phones. First antennas were made to be retractable. Of course, anytime you keep moving a small metal part, the chances of breaking it increase. Those extendable antennas were not so stable and kept breaking off. Nowadays phones are smaller and they come with three or four antennas — for GPS, for e-mail, for phone, and for texting — built directly into their backs. As a result, exposure to radio frequency radiation inside the brain is many times higher.

By 2002 the gloves were off and industry made it clear to Gandhi that they would take him on directly. Gandhi remembers being told, by an industry colleague who was once a student and friend, "If you insist on publishing these papers saying that children get more exposed than adults and saying that our test procedure is not valid, you can expect that we will not fund you."

Gandhi replied, "I am a university professor. I don't need your money."

Next industry tried to place an article by Chou critiquing Gandhi's models in the journal of which Gandhi had been editor in chief, and in which he had published dozens of articles, and asked that either his article criticizing the grounds for setting standards be removed, or that they be allowed to publish Chou's rejoinder.

Gandhi reports that "four different peer reviews of Chou's critique of my work indicated that Chou's critique of our work was 'scientific junk.'" Only when the editor of the journal balked did industry finally relent.

"Do Not Hold Directly On The Body"

Despite this success in beating back one attempt to discredit Gandhi's work, the effort to increase allowable amounts of radio frequency radiation was won on a major front. As the new chief of the standard-setting committee, Chou masterminded changes in the standards, and the committee, which now included a large majority of industry experts, issued new recommendations, ignoring Gandhi's analyses showing that these would effectively double exposures.

In fact, the real story of how much weaker current standards are, and how much higher exposures they allow into the brain, has yet to be told. Here's what we do know. Someone is getting the message somewhere. How else to explain the fact that all new manuals for all new cell phones include warnings to keep the phones away from the body? Some, like the BlackBerry, urge the distance be .98 inches, a completely impractical goal for most sensible working people. Others, like those from Finland's Nokia, say in capital letters, do not hold directly on the body. Current approaches by the IEEE calculate peak spatial-average absorption rates for safety compliance testing of cell phones based on a physical model of SAM with an added ten-millimeter plastic spacer to model what they call the pinna, formerly known as the ear. This use of a spacer actually worsens the allowed exposure considerably and assumes that the radio frequency energy absorption in the ear, which sits right next to the brain, is in fact no different from that of the legs and the arms. The next time someone tells you that your extremities are just like your brains, make sure he is not trying to sell you something.

To calculate the specific absorption rate (SAR) of phones requires knowing a few simple things. You need to know how thick the tissue is, because this determines how well radio frequency signals go through it. You need to know how big the tissue is and how much it weighs, because its mass also determines absorption, and you need to know how strong the signal is. The formula for putting this all together is pretty simple math. Without belaboring it, the absorption rate, or SAR, combines information on signal strength and the type and amount of tissue exposed.

Here's where it gets really interesting. The European approach allows the amount of mass over which radiation is averaged to be ten grams of tissue, equivalent to slightly less than an inch cube of brain cells. The U.S. standard allows a one-gram mass of tissue, which is less than a half-inch cube of brain cells. The European volume is actually three times bigger than that of the United States. The smaller the space in which you are estimating an average, the less extreme the variation in temperature will be. Obviously, using a larger volume allows more exposure overall than using a smaller one, and also means that much higher exposures can occur in selected small areas of the larger volume.

Imagine that you had a good old heavy number 10 cast iron frying pan; you've greased the pan, salted it, and you're about to cook a steak. Imagine further that you put the steak in the pan so that only half of it is actually touching the hot portion of the pan, and the other half is hanging over the side. Now, in that scenario, the average temperature might produce a perfect steak, but the reality is that the portion in the pan is going to get cooked, and the portion hanging out the side is going to remain raw. This is very reminiscent of several cautions by N. N. Taleb in *The Black Swan* — one should never depend upon the average depth when deciding whether to wade across a river. The fact that the average is four feet does not at all protect you from downing in a seven-foot-deep hole.

Thus, the logic of averaging radio frequency radiation over a larger mass of ten grams, when the brain includes many different parts of varying sensitivity in a much smaller zone, is fatally flawed.

Scientists have known for more than forty years that microwave radiation does not uniformly move through or heat anything. That's why the first microwave ovens bombed. The flow of microwave radiation is so uneven that the early ovens kept burning some parts of food and leaving other parts uncooked, because there would be hot spots with ten times higher exposure and cold spots with nearly none. The solution to microwave cooking was to put in turntables to keep rotating the food to be cooked so that the uneven hot spots would average out and become smoothly radiated. But we can't rotate our brains while we are on the cell phone.

In 1972, Allan Frey, then a young basic researcher studying medical uses of electricity, noted that exposures to radio frequency add up over time. Thus, a single exposure can produce some alteration of cells that is completely undetectable at the time and can in fact be repaired. But if the precise same area gets tweaked over and over again, repair may not happen as easily or at all. If hot spots do form in very tiny segments of the brain, and form repeatedly, then over time such impacts may not be fixable. Of course, because the brain feels no sensation directly, anyone repeatedly exposed to such microscopic damage will not be aware of it at the time.

In fact, modelers tell us that for hot spots in our own brains, SAR levels within half-inch cubes of small volumes of tissue can be 10-fold higher than those measured by the current big-guy SAM dummy model. Further, even with the SAM approach, if a child's smaller head is used, the SAR can be 2.5-fold larger. Anyone smaller than SAM, which is most of us, will receive a much larger SAR exposure, and because the volume is so high it comes nowhere close to measuring potential tissue damage.

Since 2004, the IEEE standard has effectively ignored two undeniable facts: One size does not fit all and the brain is not one consistent density. The greater vulnerability of children is not merely a topic of concern to brain modelers, but has affected policy makers in many modern nations. In 2001, a commission of the Royal College of Physicians, chaired by Sir William Stewart, issued this report:

> *If there are currently unrecognized adverse health effects from the use of mobile phones, children may be more vulnerable because of their developing nervous system,* the greater absorption of energy in the tissues of the head *(paragraph 4.37), and a longer lifetime of exposure. In line with our precautionary approach, at this time, we believe that the widespread use of mobile phones by children for nonessential calls should be discouraged. We also recommend that the mobile phone industry should refrain from promoting the use of mobile phones by children (paragraphs 6.89 and 6.90).*

Another Brainstorm

For a decade, Alan Marks, a savvy real estate analyst and developer, had been acting strangely. His wife of close to thirty years and his adult children barely spoke to him any longer. Normally a natural comic, he became morose, prone to rages and erratic behavior. He would suddenly yell about something, forget where he had placed any number of important objects, and go through periods of disabling, deep depression. A string of psychiatrists prescribed various medications and much family counseling. He was diagnosed as bipolar. None asked about his habitual use of cell phones.

The night before his youngest child's graduation from college, May 6, 2008, as he slept Marks began to fling his fists and legs wildly and could not stop. His neck arched back and he began to shudder and shake. His mouth opened to let out deep guttural sounds. His terrified wife, Ellie, called 911. Marks was having a grand mal seizure. In the emergency room, Ellie learned that Marks had a golfball-size tumor in the glial cells of his brain, right where he had held a variety of cell phones for close to two decades — more than ten thousand hours overall. Alan and Ellie Marks are on a mission to tell their story.

"If only someone had told me that holding the phone right next to my head could give me a brain tumor, I would not be dealing with my death sentence. I would have done what I am doing now, using an earpiece or a speakerphone," Marks told me one day, when we met to talk about his situation.

"I am angry. My life is going to end because nobody was paying attention to what this device could do to my brain. It's not fair that industry can make a product that can rob a man of his life, and they have no responsibility to warn us about this.

"If there had been a warning twenty-seven years ago, I still would have used a cell phone," he said, "but I wouldn't have put it to my head. That's the issue. People are not being warned that the way they use cell phones now can kill them later."

"When you put that phone to your head, you are unknowingly playing Russian roulette," Marks told a hearing in Maine that was considering warning labels on cell phones.

"It's too late for me, but it's not too late for my children or yours," Marks urged.

And Another

Mindy Brown is woman who knows firsthand what the Markses are saying. She watched her tall, athletic, strapping husband become a bedridden, swollen-headed invalid within two years. As defensive coach for Fresno State, and the sort of man people had a hard time saying no to, Dan Brown worked his phone relentlessly, as he traveled the state recruiting top football talent. He used to joke that he was frying his brain, because his ear would become so hot. In fact, the sort of heat that the ear feels may have nothing to do with the fact that invisible radio frequency signals can create hot spots and disturb cells inside the brain inches below the area of the phone where antennas are buried. The brain itself cannot feel heat or pain. By the time the skin at the skull is hot, much more has happened below the surface deep within the brain. Over time some hot spots never heal and lose their ability to control abnormal growth. These microscopic sites of damage may become seeds from which brain tumors can generate.

As he went through hours of surgery, radiation, and chemotherapy, Coach Brown knew his chances were slim. He tried keeping it light, offering up his usual patter of jokes and one-liners. He asked Mindy, his high school sweetheart and wife, as he lay unable to move just hours before his death, what he could do for her. "Please, please," she pleaded. "Please don't die. Don't leave me."

He replied, "I'm sorry, I just cannot control that anymore. But you can do something for me."

"Yes," she responded. "What's that?"

The coach urged, "Just make sure that they know, that the world hears what happened to me."

Mindy is keeping her word. So is her son Larry, at twenty-four the oldest of their six children. At the hearing of the legislative committee reviewing a bill to put warning labels on phones in Maine, in March 2010, Larry asked a question that no one could answer.

Holding up a copy of tiny print found in cell phone packaging, he read it aloud. "'Warning, do not hold the phone on the body.'

"Why are phone companies putting these warnings into their new phones today?" Larry wondered. "Is there something else they are not telling us?"

Those committee members who were paying attention were caught off-guard by this question. It was clear that some of them did not believe what they had heard. They asked to see the thin and crinkled piece of paper that Larry held up. They passed it around and saw that Larry was right. There it was in black and white.

Do you know anyone who uses a cell phone holding it an inch from her ear?

It's quite likely that the phones that Marks and Brown used in the 1990s complied with the SAM-based standards. Remember, these presume that calls last six minutes — after that time it was then believed that tissue could start to heat up. In fact, standards for cell phones used by Coach Brown and Alan Marks were set when few people owned phones. They have not been changed since.

Marks is five feet ten. Brown was six feet tall. Neither of them quite measured up to SAM. Yet the phones that they used all had radiation releases based on the bigger brain and shorter calls that SAM would have made.

The new warnings found deep inside the packaging of all modern phones today use this same big-guy model talking for six minutes. Today three out of every four twelve-year-olds have a phone, as do half of all ten-year-olds. Their heads are obviously getting a lot more exposure than what SAM would get, if he ever were real. And few of them will ever see the fine-print warning labels that come with more and more phones today. But that could soon change.

6

THE DOKTOR WHO DANCED
WITH THE DEVIL

*The desire to tell the truth is therefore only one condition for being an intellectual.
The other is courage, readiness to carry on rational inquiry to wherever it may lead.*

~Paul Baran

Herr Professor Doktor Franz Adlkofer was flummoxed. For close to two decades, this tall, powerful man was someone everyone wanted to know. Adlkofer had the one thing on which all scientists depend — lots of ready money. His job was to dispense millions in euros to scientists around the globe investigating one of the most profitable gaseous mixtures — tobacco smoke. So long as the questions they were asked to study seemed like serious science, professors found ways to accept tobacco moneys, hire more research assistants, and publish their research. The urbane, multilingual Adlkofer was used to being listened to.

He was not used to being marginalized.

A frequent spring time visitor to Greece, he had ambled through the harbor streets of Piraeus, just outside Athens, many times. Hewing to the cooler shaded sidewalks of the big old buildings at Platia

119

Karaiskaki near the bus station across from the Metro, he would stay out of the sweltering heat. At the start of his visit to his Greek home, he bought tickets on the regular ferry to the island of Paros. He avoided the street hustlers on Nikis Street who sell gullible tourists fake Rolexes and pricey tickets for cruises when all they want is a simple ferry fare.

Surrounded by rich green vines and gardens of olives, oranges, and pomegranates, Paros rests on cool, white marble rising out of the sea. Adlkofer's home, like most of those on this Cycladic island, was built with flat roofs, thick whitewashed walls, and bright blue painted doors, window frames, and shutters. Paros offered a safe, solid haven and cool, steady sea breezes.

At the beginning of the summer in 2008, the air full of the scent of flowers, Adlkofer was preparing to take a string of slow car ferries that would bring him back to Germany. First, his wife and he had sailed on the ferry back to Pireaus. From that bustling port they had to drive the serpentine coastal road to Patras, where three months earlier they had booked the slow overnight boat to Venice. Adlkofer knew that, like most of the seaside roads of Greece, the road to Patras had no guardrails. Every month or so, someone drives over the edge. But he'd planned the journey meticulously and made the drive without incident.

Just a half hour after his arrival in Patras, at about ten o'clock, Adlkofer was about to board and secure space for his car. The late sunset had just given way to a glistening moonlit sea.

But the darkness that hit Adlkofer as he was about to set foot on the ferryboat ramp would shatter his end-of-summer reverie. While looking out at the Aegean, taking in the salty air, the muffled but persistent ring of his cell phone startled him. He had not remembered turning it on. He rummaged for it in his hand luggage, unsure of where it was. He thought that whoever was calling probably had the wrong number. But he hastened to grab the phone to be sure that nothing important was wrong. As he pressed the speaker button, he heard the distraught voice of his senior colleague Herr Professor Doktor Hugo Rüdiger. Blood drained from his face as he listened. His decades-long, distinguished scientific career was kaput. Adlkofer had been accused of fraud — the kiss of death for any scientist. He had just stepped onto the ferryboat deck but could not move.

The Dance

For years, as the chief of tobacco research in Germany, Adlkofer had danced with the devil. He had produced dazzling technical research that kept executives at Reemtsma, Sturm-Zigaretten, and other German tobacco firms confident of their strategy of investing in complicated scientific work. The complexity of the science became a kind of shield. We don't precisely understand how the more than four thousand compounds in tobacco smoke work, they reasoned. We just know that combined they cause an enormous risk to the health of people. Therefore, let's make the products less harmful.

Of course, Adlkofer himself never smoked and never would. But like many scientists who grew up in postwar Germany, he knew a good opportunity when he saw it. Adlkofer had held sway over the expansive German tobacco research empire because he managed to have it both ways: He told the truth where he found it, and what he found about the way that tobacco affected living cells was often more complicated than convenient. For a long while his work did dovetail with commercial interests, but ultimately it did not.

When Adlkofer spoke about all this to me one hot summer day in Vienna, he was determined to convince me that becoming the chief of the scientific department of the German Industry Association had been merely a sensible career option. We sat outside the nineteenth-century wedding cake structure of the Hotel Regina, on a terrace surrounded by tired-looking palm trees, drinking mineral water. Occasional breezes cooled the humid ninety-degree temperature. Even the ants moved slowly across the granite pavers beneath our feet.

Adlkofer explained that early in his professional life, dazzling technologies that deciphered the most basic operations of cells enthralled him. He had spent hours riveted by images of the engines of cellular life — mitochondria — that fueled all growth. He longed to spend a lifetime exploring the exquisite complexity of living matter. "In 1975, in Berlin when I finished my medical training in endocrinology and internal medicine, there were no jobs for me, none at all. Prized posts in academic medicine were almost inherited, passed down from one mentor to another. You had to wait for someone to die to get one.

"I had a wife and young family and had achieved some distinction academically. All of a sudden an invitation from industry arrived. I was surprised when I met people in the tobacco research group who were totally different from the people who work with tobacco today. These were not the slimy bastards I'd expected, but honorable people with what looked like important questions. Germany had its own cigarette industry. The bosses of this industry suffered personally. They got it. They knew that their product was killing people."

As he talked, I sat with my arms folded, feeling skeptical.

Adlkofer flashed a tight smile that told me to hold my fire. He took a sip of sparkling water and went on.

"The Germans believed there simply had to be a way to make smoking safer, they really did. So they went about collecting a lot of scientists around them who would advise them about how to do this. They needed someone to organize the scientists who understood the work and who could work alongside them and get things done."

Even in his seventies, Adlkofer has a commanding, confident air. Standing more than six feet tall, he has a large forehead and an assertive voice. He comes from a family of organizers. His father survived as a prisoner of war in Italy directing inmates to carry out sanitation projects. As a young man, Adlkofer had served as an officer in the German army on various education efforts. He retains the demeanor and the temperament of someone used to giving orders and having them followed.

With my chin in my hands, my elbows on the table, I'm sure I didn't look convinced. I wasn't.

"I can appreciate that you find all this hard to believe, but I was given what I thought was the chance of a lifetime. My research council on smoking and health had the leading scientists in the medical field simply because tobacco money could provide funding when there was frankly nothing else available. Our German bosses believed that there had to be a real chance that their product could be improved. They really, really believed this. The Americans never did.

"All of a sudden, I was working with the highest ranking scientists in the entire world. We had enough money to do so."

He paused, looked up, and moved both his open hands over the tabletop, then thudded his palms onto the table and repeated, "We had a lot of money."

I nodded hesitantly as he continued.

"This went on for years. Our funds supported conferences, graduate students, postdocs, publications, and lots of trips to attend meetings and even issue special issues of journals based on select conferences — all the usual sorts of scientific work that people still struggle to support."

In the decades following the war, the sense that science could be value-free and open had been hailed as the mark of a democratic society. The philosopher Karl Popper argued in *The Open Society and Its Enemies* — his two-volume work published during World War II — that a truly free marketplace of ideas was central to democracy. In his essays Herbert Marcuse, an intellectual father of sixties student revolutionaries, countered that only science that served political and economic justice would prove worthwhile. Germany's population continued to reel from the corruption of science and technology under the Nazis, and wanted to believe in the neutrality of good, honest scientific investigation. In such a culture, where research money came from to support science might reasonably be seen as unimportant.

The Free University of Berlin, where Adlkofer completed his medical training, was free but not much of a university in the early 1970s. Still isolated by the Soviet Union's "iron curtain," West Berlin remained more or less dependent on the air bridge the Allies had set up decades before. New graduates, like Adlkofer, from East Berlin, were treated as though they were tainted by the communism that pervaded the region. Encircled by walls, guns, and tanks within sight of the rubble of East Berlin, young researchers had limited resources and avenues for advancement.

Those living within university walls, real or imagined, tend to maintain a cocky disinterest in practical matters. Freud once said, clearly referring to himself, that those who become scientists tend to have the habits of mind that make them appear far older and more serious as children. A photo of the five-year-old Sigmund in the Freud Museum in Vienna shows a suited and bespectacled young boy seated at a huge desk, looking like a junior professor. As adults scientists manage to retain the bold curiosity, playfulness, bravado, sense of immortality, and indifference to doubt of the young. In my meetings and correspondence with Adlkofer, I found the symmetry uncanny. Here was a man who looked like central casting's version of a somber gray eminence with the audacity of an adolescent.

To the annoyance of his tobacco industry patrons, by 1992 Adlkofer began to make a simple argument. We know that tobacco is killing people and we know that nicotine becomes a hard habit to kick because of what it does to the brain. But if we can find a way to isolate or remove the most damaging components of tobacco, we can halve the toll of lung cancer and let people smoke in a safer manner that will also be highly profitable.

The tobacco industry had a problem. They had started out dispensing funds generously throughout the impoverished university system to generate public confusion and buy scientific goodwill. There were growing complaints that they couldn't control Adlkofer. After all, like the defiant adolescent who never quite grows out of the role of provocateur, he had repeatedly produced a body of work showing that smoking was a public health catastrophe.

Adlkofer was ready to move on but perhaps not as ready as the tobacco industry was for him to do so. The deal they cut was simple. In 1993, Adlkofer got start-up money to become head of a new foundation — the Verum (the Latin noun for "truth") Foundation — focusing on narrow scientific questions, devising models and methods for studying how the brain responded to various cues from the environment. It would be funded by tobacco money for several years. The scientific truths that Verum began to uncover would turn out to have a much longer life.

At the time, antitobacco activists smelled a rat. Watch out, they said, he is just going to distract people from realizing how bad tobacco really is.

Not surprisingly, Adlkofer started at Verum detailing the addictive effects of nicotine on the brain. But within two years Verum had begun broader studies of proteins that can affect the speed with which the brain thinks, hears, or reacts. The research moved from dissecting nicotine to identifying other agents that harm nerve cells and underlie Alzheimer's, Parkinson's, and other devastating syndromes of a degenerating nervous system like autism. The Verum-funded researchers knew that, like cancer, most cases of these diseases do not come about because of who your parents are but because of what happens to you after you are born. While degenerative diseases of the brain have a range of names and limited types of treatments, they share one thing: All include strange abnormalities and clumping of proteins.

In securing support for his ambitious neuroscience research program, Adlkofer played scientific double agent. To the original tobacco industry funders, he was adding legitimacy to their enterprise and moving on and out of their hair by taking their money to do credible and basic work on mysteries of the brain. To tobacco critics, he was ending the pretense that there was any way to make tobacco smoking healthy and switching to other even more esoteric work.

As the twenty-first century began, Verum and Adlkofer achieved a major coup. The European Union awarded the REFLEX group of laboratory collaborators that Adlkofer led five million dollars to study electromagnetic signals, including the sort that come from cell phones. Might these affect our brains? Fundamentally, Adlkofer didn't think this was possible. He knew that most scientists felt that low levels of radio frequency radiation could not have any impact on neurons. Still, people were beginning to ask what the new cell phone technology might do to their brains and bodies. And this was the kind of question he had devoted his life to investigating.

In 1993, fewer than 1 percent of all Americans used cell phones. That same year, the family of Susan Reynard of Tampa, Florida, filed a lawsuit claiming that her deadly brain tumor had been caused by her unusually heavy use of one of those older clunky cell phones. Within a week of her widower David's appearance on *Larry King Live* discussing the case, stock prices for phone companies and service providers dropped about 10 percent. The filing of a lawsuit alleging that any technology produces a serious health problem is not easily undertaken. Such a suit usually only happens after attorneys and experts have concluded that there is merit to the matter and that they are willing to put up the time and money to pursue it. Other claims soon followed.

By 1997, Congressman Edward Markey, chair of the House Subcommittee on Telecommunications and the Internet, expressed serious doubts about whether the widely touted multi-million-dollar industry-governmental partnership to study cell phones and health with the Cellular Telecommunications Industry Association (CTIA) could produce reliable and independent results. The congressman called for a firewall to be created to assure that the research was carried out without improper influence. As a result, the Wireless Technology Research Limited Liability Company (WTR) came into existence. The industry was not comfortable with all this public attention coming just as the marketing of cell phones was about to take off. It seems likely they saw the new body as a good hedge. The head of the twenty-five-million-dollar WTR was a lawyer-scientist, George Carlo, who had defended the chemical industry when it was under fire for dioxin pollution. By 2000, more than a hundred million phones were in use in the United States and more cases alleging that brain tumors had been caused by cell phones had been filed. The very existence of a large ongoing research program provided a sort of sop to those who expressed any concerns: Trust us. We are so concerned about the issue that we are spending lots of money studying it.

Adlkofer recalls, "Before we began our own study of cell phones, Verum had supported the work of Michael Repacholi at the World Health Organization. Repacholi had a sophisticated view of the issue. Let's just say he was inclined toward the idea that we needed to find out if electromagnetic signals pose a health risk." "So," I said, "Repacholi knowing your tobacco history thought of you as someone who was, shall we say, a bit flexible?"

Adlkofer took this as an affront. "Well, of course, any sensible scientist knows that if you could actually make tobacco less toxic, that would have been a good thing. But that was not what we focused on then. As to radio frequencies, what little I knew about the topic told me that it simply had to be safe. We hypothesized that if we were to run the studies on radio frequency radiation using live cell cultures in our laboratory and did not see anything happening at this cellular or molecular level, we could conclude it would be a waste of money to do any further research. Our a priori opinion was that we would find no health effects at all from radio frequency radiation."

A New Finding?

In 2000, Adlkoker's team started the REFLEX project within the fifth European Framework Programme. Under carefully controlled conditions, Verum researchers worked with two different types of cells. Human cells and animal cells taken from rodents were each subjected to levels of radio frequency radiation found in cell phones. Exposed and unexposed cells were then run through an array of laboratory exams to see if exposed cells looked any different in how they communicated, healed, or died. Groups of scientists working at a dozen different institutions across Europe were examining whether radio frequency signals had any impact on the complex acid making up the genetic materials of all cells — our DNA.

Adlkofer says, "After several months of research, I got the first information that there is something strange going on. It looked like radio frequency was damaging cells. So the first thing we did was to look at the equipment to see if there was some problem. Our idea was that this equipment we were using must not be not good enough. Our equipment belongs in a museum. I just did not believe these results could be true."

Problems with measuring equipment can create all sorts of strange findings. Many scientists scrounge for funds for their labs to get reliable microscopes, centrifuges, and good old-fashioned refrigerators. Some become adept at shopping at bankruptcy sales for spare parts. Adlkofer was in a different league. He didn't need to worry about such things.

"We had lots of money, so we went out and got brand-new equipment. We set it all up carefully. And we ran the work again, exposing the cells to RF and looking inside at their DNA. And again we found the very same effects. The DNA from the exposed cells looked sick. We saw an increase in DNA strand breaks. Not just in one of our laboratories, but in two separate facilities, in Charité in Berlin, also in Vienna. We were astonished."

The cell phone industry was also stunned. It had never imagined that one of its own — so to speak — a man whose reputation had been cut by working with the tobacco industry — might prove to be difficult to control. The REFLEX team had followed all the rules. First they issued a number of posters and papers explaining the results to scientific conferences full of intense, earnest young and old scientists eager to be seen as on the cutting edge of various specialties. Then they repeated the same tests and got the same results in different laboratories. Finally, they submitted the work for publication and it went through the usual process of review, where experts try to pick apart the interpretation. Having survived these gauntlets, the REFLEX results finally appeared as a series of publications, all showing an increase in profound disruption of genetic material — DNA strand breaks. The teams also consistently found increases in a type of damage called micronuclei, which proves the existence of serious genetic defects leading down the path to cancer. The normal nucleus at the center of healthy cells contains all that is needed to keep things under control. Deformed copies of the nucleus, micronuclei, demonstrate that this cell will not be able to continue its normal life.

This was yet another scientific finding that displeased the cell phone industry. Nearly ten years after Lai and Singh's comet assay and its demonstration, and forty years after the Office of Naval Research had sponsored studies finding biological impacts that few ever heard of, here was even more incontrovertible evidence that DNA could be damaged by radio frequency of precisely the sort used by the latest generation of phones — both 2G and 3G. This kind and extent of DNA damage became a very inconvenient fact of life — one that could not be allowed to stand unchallenged. These results were seen by the industry as a major public relations problem requiring a strong and swift response: Deny that the analysis could possibly be valid. Attack those who did the work.

And secure others to come up with studies that look just like those you don't like that manage to reach opposite conclusions.

A Buried Finding

Adlkofer's team did not know much about the details of Lai and Singh's work from 1996, which had pretty much been dismissed after more and more studies were soon published that failed to reproduce the same results. At that point, few working in the field had heard about extensive work carried out nearly half a century earlier by Frey and others — long before cell phones had been commercialized — showing that radio frequency radiation could break the brain barrier and interfere with other biological membranes. In 1960, when the navy was forging improved types of radar, neuroscientist Allan Frey, then with Cornell University's General Electric Advanced Electronics Center, had become curious about the impact on the nervous system of electromagnetic fields moving at the speed of light. A fellow who had been tasked with measuring signals released by radar stations told Frey that he could "hear" radar.

At the time, psychiatrists treated people who claimed to hear radio signals inside their heads as delusional schizophrenics. Frey was understandably skeptical. But this radar technician seemed perfectly sane. He was. When Frey traveled to the radar station near Syracuse, New York, to listen for himself, he heard the same strange humming sound as well.

When we met in Annapolis in the spring of 2010 to discuss this work, Frey explained that, in the effort to ramp up American science capacity during the Cold War, he had been one of those chosen to receive extraordinary resources to explore basic scientific questions. "I was frankly just curious about lots of things back then and I had the freedom to explore basic science questions because the Office of Naval Research gave me unrestricted support. So I went with this fellow to the station where he worked. Sure enough, I heard a sound that I knew was not going through my ears but echoing inside my head, a kind of low soft sibilant *Zzzzipppp. Zzzzipppp, zzzzippp.*"

"How could you be sure where it was coming from?" I asked. "I made a kind of crude shield out of a metal screen. I knew that metal would block microwave signals of radar. Whenever I held this screen between his head and where the radar was coming from, the sound would disappear. When I removed the screen, the sound would return. I tried it myself and the same thing happened."

By the end of this visit, Frey was convinced that the hearing nerve was resonating in some way with the radar beam. Frey also realized that the sounds that were being heard were not coming from conventional sound waves that moved externally through air, hitting the eardrum and moving up the acoustic nerve to the brain to register as noise. In fact, the hum was being produced within the brain itself, which is why blocking the radar blocked the sound. This meant that electromagnetic waves from radar directly reached nerve cells within the brain and created tiny vibrating fields. The capacity of electromagnetic fields to cause the brain to hear sounds stunned neurobiologists. During World War II, men working close to radar equipment had also reported what became known as the microwave auditory effect — later dubbed the Frey effect for the man who first reported it in the scientific literature.

The ability of microwave signals to produce sound within the brain stunned the neuroscience community. But the Frey effect remained little known outside of a small community of scientists and was not known to

Adlkofer or other scientists who undertook basic studies on the impact of radio frequency on brain biology nearly three decades later.

In the days before the Internet, it was not at all hard to keep collaboration between the Department of Defense and universities under wraps.

The sheer complexity of bioelectromagnetics — as the field Frey helped to invent came to be known — made it easy. Few of us then or now have more than the most rudimentary grasp of electricity, where it comes from, how it's made, and what it can do to our health. To most of us electricity is that thing that happens when we turn on the light switch or plug in the hair dryer. As Frey's work evolved — and its implications became clear at least to some — those funding his efforts at the Office of Naval Research offered him the sort of friendly advice that no scientist could afford to ignore.

Frey determined that the carrier wave of 1,900 megahertz — precisely the same wavelength used by many cell phones today — interacted with the voices and noises carried on that wave, the data, in some important ways. Inject a mouse with blue dye in its blood — something a curious scientist did earlier in the last century — and the entire body and all of the organs turn blue, with one exception. The brain remains pink-gray. The brilliant Russian biochemist Lina Solomonova Stern theorized in the 1920s, when she first did this work, that the brain is protected from taking in poisons or contaminants that get into the bloodstream by what is called the blood-brain barrier. By the 1960s the truth of this view had been made clear when electron microscopy traced the movement of injected dye through the bloodstream. Even when toxic blue agents enter the blood, this barrier will block them from entering the brain.

Frey soon found a way to change that. He showed that radio frequency signals — just like those from today's cell phones — opened up this normally closed barrier. Frey first injected a dark dye into the bloodstream of standard laboratory Sprague-Dawley white rats. Then he exposed these rats to pulsed microwave signals. Within a few minutes the brains of the injected rats that had been microwaved began to turn bright yellow-green, signaling that the blood-brain barrier had been breached. Brain cells need all the protection they can get to work normally. Frey's studies were reported in the *Annals of the New York Academy of Sciences* in 1975. Adlkofer had never seen them.

The Frey Effect Besieged

In 1974, Om P. Gandhi had just started working in this field as a consultant to Walter Reed Army Medical Center. In 1973, he had been offered funding to conduct research with the military on radio frequency for four months, so he left his young family and worked from August to December in Reed's barracks laboratory.

"One thing I studied was this so-called auditory phenomenon that everybody had heard about from Frey. People were scratching their heads about this. I said we could set this up and see if this was real or not. We used a horn antenna with pulsed power. With continuous wave you get nothing. But with jagged, pulsed signals like those that power today's smart phones, we could produce this sound. "Bill Guy and the fellows that asked me to study this were well supported by the Defense Department and frankly doubted what Frey had reported. So I sat there myself and I could hear that sound. So could some of the young men who were working with us. As you changed the pulse rate to higher and higher rates per second, you could hear the tones change as well. But it was mostly a kind of low drone or *hummmmmmmmmm, hummmmmmmm, hummmmmmmm.*

"Of course, Guy had suggested the experiment because he did not believe it. As I think back on it, they were determined to find some way to indicate that the Frey effect had been an artifact — not a real thing — but something that happens in an experiment because of the way things were set up. At the time, I was just getting started in this field and did not understand that there were people out there who simply did not want to believe that microwavelike radiation could have any biological impacts. To show them that there was something real and physical going on, I crumpled up some paper and did the study again. When it was exposed to pulsed radio frequency signals, the paper would rattle. I crinkled up some aluminum foil, and it also would shake. Everybody could hear this sound made by the radio frequency radiation reverberating, because the quivering foil or paper made sounds of their own when the radiation hit.

"Although I was a senior professor in microwave engineering, I was a newcomer in the field of biological impacts of electrical matters, so I published this as simply showing that Frey had been right and let it go. A year or so later, Guy, who was senior to me in the field, decided that I had been wrong and that a thermoelastic (heat-based) wave had caused this sound. Guy was an electrical engineer who was pretty powerful and influential at the time. And I knew better than to tussle with him. He had money and clout and held sway over everyone in the field then and for a long time afterwards."

Despite the work of Frey, Lai, Gandhi, and others, along with Adlkofer's confirmation that microwave-like radiation from cell phones induces biological damage, the science continues to be debated. In many instances what looks like refutations of research turn out to be poor imitations. Over the past several years, Lin, an ICNIRP member, has produced a number of papers appearing to refute Frey's work on the ability of pulsed microwave radiation to induce sounds in the brain. In point of fact, Lin's critiques ignore Frey's primary paper on the topic that appeared in *Science* magazine in 1979. Using holography, an exquisitely sensitive technique that does not destroy tissue, Frey found that microwave pulses do not create motion in soft tissue. Lin's studies finding a signal on the auditory nerve resulted from an experimental artifact. The tiny electrode assembly he used to "detect sound" actually produced it. When Frey invented and patented (for the Office of Naval Research) a special, nonintrusive electrode, he was able to show that the creation of sound in the brain does result from the low-intensity microwave signals, quite like those released by cell phones today.

In his most recent critique of Frey, Lin ignores Frey's Science paper completely. Instead, he cites five of Frey's other papers, giving the appearance of thoroughness. Frey comments on this highly selective reading of his work: "This sort of thing has always been done by the 'no hazard establishment people' since the beginning, and has misled scientists and the public. . . ."

Frey recalls that some of the studies purporting to show that Frey's work on the blood-brain barrier were wrong, did no such thing. "One group claimed to repeat our studies and find nothing. But instead of injecting fluorescent dye into the artery where it could circulate like I did, they injected it into the abdomen, waited five minutes, killed the animals, and found no evidence that the dye had reached the brain. Of course not."

To this day, Frey does not think highly of Guy.

"Bill Guy was an interesting man, an electrical engineer, who didn't know a thing about biology. The Air Force experts in aviation medicine used to pour lots of money into him. When Bill did his big five-million-dollar study of cancer in rodents exposed to microwaves, I raised questions about the analysis. They had actually thrown out brain tumors! Of course, they found no evidence of an effect.

"Once when Bill and I were over in the Soviet Union we met at a lab to have a little discussion about the microwave stuff. We were sitting around a table — about eighteen of us, including Soviet scientists. This woman who headed the experimental lab studying health and microwaves turned to Bill and said, 'Dr. Guy, tell me about the work being done in your lab.' He sort of sat there and sat there, with his head down. He turned to me and said, 'Allan, would you tell them about the work being done in my group?' as he didn't really know what was being done regarding biological work."

One of the studies done in Guy's lab was an investigation of cancer in animals exposed to radio frequency radiation. The first results showed that microwave-like radiation increased cancer in animals. Gandhi and three others have told me this story. The reported finding of a significantly increased cancer risk with microwave exposure is one that the military funders of that work did not want to have seen in print. And it wasn't.

Frey and Gandhi today are at the ends of their careers. They understand that there was a lot of pressure exerted on researchers at the time to stay away from studies that suggested that radio frequency radiation had biological impacts of any kind. Radar installations and satellite systems were being set up around the country. Research suggesting that these required any special handling was not welcome during the height of the Cold War — a point that Paul Brodeur thoroughly documented in his book *The Zapping of America*, published in 1977, and serialized in The *New Yorker* that same year.

In response to Brodeur's writings, the government activated a Committee on Man and Radiation (COMAR), headed up by a Veterans Administration psychologist, Don Justesen. COMAR mounted a major public relations campaign to rebut and discredit Brodeur's conclusions that certain exposures to microwave radiation could cause genetic damage, blindness, and changes in behavior. In reaching his views about these dangers, Brodeur interviewed dozens of Defense Department researchers and relied in part on some of Frey's work. Frey believed that the New Yorker critique that COMAR prepared included a number of misrepresentations about his own research.

When confronted about these misstatements, Justesen told Frey that the COMAR critique had been a draft that would be revised further and had not been widely distributed. Frey knew this was not true. He had been given a copy of the rebuttal that had in fact been submitted to *The New Yorker* for publication, but had been rejected. Even today, some three decades later, Frey is appalled by two facts:

"The guys heading up COMAR just did not understand biology. What happened here was a naked use of power to try to discredit what had been basic scientific work because it did not comport with what those funding the work wanted at the time."

At one point, in 1978, Frey was invited to a major meeting ostensibly set up to review his work that was billed as an effort to reach consensus in the field. It proved to be no such thing. Rather, Bill Guy and others came and presented studies that the Department of Energy had funded that had been designed to show that, contrary to Frey, microwave radiation did not affect the blood-brain barrier, did not affect the formation of cataracts, nor genes of living tissue. The existence of conflicting science was used in a magical way. Frey saw that the margins of the draft report had contained a penciled query regarding the advice that there was no need to study the blood-brain barrier: "Do you really want to say this?"

In his summary of this meeting, Justesen, who himself was not an expert in the field, basically wrote that since there was conflict among scientists on the issue, there was no problem. And there was also no need for further research.

Today, Gandhi looks back on these efforts with a different perspective.

"At the time I did the work on the Frey effect, and even later when I showed that brain models needed to be changed, a number of people put a lot of effort into trying to discredit findings they did not like. In our field, half of the people have made up their minds that there are no effects and they tend to get support from industry and the military. About a quarter of the people think that there are effects everywhere at any level at all, and they tend to work without any government support."

"What about you?" I asked. "Where do you fit in?"

Gandhi paused a moment and said, "The rest of us who are neither doubters nor true believers think maybe there are some important effects that need to be controlled and that microwave radiation plays some very valuable roles in our society today. Microwave technology has made remarkable improvements in many parts of our society from aviation to medicine. But we certainly need to find out how to use it as safely as possible and not deny that it can be harmful. As long as the funds were available, back then we did the work. But a lot of people in this field had made up their minds, and many of those who did, like Bill Guy and Don Justesen, got the most money and basically set the stage for what could and could not be done for years. Of course, now, there is no money for independent research at all.

"So long as I stayed out of the biology of radio frequency radiation, I was able to find funds for my students and me to study electrical engineering. But in the United States the Bioelectromagnetics Society has died off, because most people in positions of power decided that there can be no biological effects. Of course, there can't be effects if we can't get funding to study them. Anytime there is evidence of an effect, there are many others brought in to show that there is nothing."

Gandhi has repeatedly provided one message on all this. In the United States the standards for radio frequency radiation that he helped to write were set up long before cell phones were in wide use, based in large part on work that Gandhi and his students carried out in the 1970s through the early 1990s. Those standards have not been changed since then.

In decades past Defense Department researchers carried out an entirely separate line of inquiry on radio frequency. They sought to build new weapons and ways of deactivating land mines. Scientists had long known that pulsed microwave signals could kill rats by stopping their breathing and could also produce potentially lethal blood clots. In a dramatic demonstration of the power of radio frequency in 1985, the Spanish neuroscientist José Delgado used a pulsed signal sent deep into the brain to stop a charging bull. Prospects for using such signals for a variety of other purposes — ranging from destruction to construction to medicine — seemed limitless.

Backs to the Future

Adlkofer didn't know about Frey or his studies until he and I met almost forty years later. After his encounters with those who urged him to move on to other work, Frey's efforts became one of those little known developments in the history of science.

When efforts were started to undermine the findings of the REFLEX project, Adlkofer recognized them for what they were. Perhaps it was hubris, but he had not ever imagined that he would find himself subject to the same sort of blunt attacks that the tobacco industry had carried out for years against its own critics. He had a strange sort of self-understanding throughout his career. He recognized that the tobacco industry on some level didn't really care about what he was doing. They were buying complexity as a way to stave off regulatory action and responsibility. So long as his own work was truly independent and scientifically grounded, he felt no moral compunction about carrying it out.

But the cell phone story was different. Adlkofer had grandchildren and had reached a moment in his career when he was in the position to retire to a pleasant life. But he could not leave in disgrace, because he knew something that others did not. He knew that the work carried out on DNA damage caused by radio frequency radiation was firmly established. He suspected foul play behind the swift and unusually public efforts to charge him with fraud.

Just the accusation of fraud often ends a scientist's career. As the REFLEX results began to appear, a major public relations firm in

Germany was brought in to respond for the cell phone industry and cloud what Verum had in fact determined. The German cell phone industry's lobbying group — Forschungsgemeinschaft Funk — led by Dr. Gerd Friedrich, dismissed the results as being flawed.

Meanwhile, Professor Alexander Lerchl at the private Jacobs University in Bremen wrote a letter to the rector of the University of Vienna alleging that the REFLEX statistics were wrong, demanding that the data be reviewed and that the paper be withdrawn from the scientific literature. Lerchl sent similar demands to the editors of the journal *Mutation Research* and *International Archives of Occupational and Environmental Health*, which had published the results, and to the authors as well, asking them to print a retraction. In sending this letter, Lerchl failed to note one important detail — he was not merely a concerned independent scientist, as he represented himself to be. For years, Lerchl had received generous funding from a joint industry-government program. From 2002 to 2008, the Deutsches Mobilfunk Forschungsprogramm (German Mobile Phone Research Program) provided 8.5 million euros, matched by government funds, to various research groups all over Europe. Lerchl himself got more than one million euros to carry out five different projects on the biological impacts of radio frequency. His work has been unerringly consistent — none of it has found any biological impact of radio frequency on health. Vodafone Foundation — created by the world's largest cell phone company — is also a major supporter of this university. Lerchl became chair of the commission responsible for the protection of people from nonionizing radiation, within the German national committee SSK (Strahlensschutzkommission).

The Blood-Brain Barrier Revisited

When someone who has spent years working for and getting rich off of tobacco money suddenly presents himself as a champion of truth, well, how credible is he?

"What did you think industry would do when you produced this work showing that cell signals could disrupt basic biology? After all, you had been one of the tobacco boys for quite a while," I asked him.

"Of course, some people may not trust me. But what happened to us after we published our findings showing DNA damage from radio frequency radiation certainly was not the sort of thing that happens to those who are in the inner circle of power. After our results started to come out showing that radio frequency radiation damaged cells, first industry ignored us. Then they decided to take us on, and they did so in what turned out to be a pretty dirty fashion."

Dirty or not, the same European Union that had provided groups Adlkofer headed with more than twenty million euros, mostly for research on what can turn our healthy nervous systems sick, decided not to renew the work on cell phone radiation. And it did so — basically pulling the plug midstream — while Adlkofer was in the middle of determining what radio frequency signals did to basic biology. There are always budgetary concerns and other factors in political decisions such as this, but it does seem that those unhappy with these results made sure that funding would end quickly. Under normal circumstances a loss of millions of dollars in funding for a big, complicated project would have been a death sentence. But this project was exceptional. Adlkofer was not accustomed to running out of money for any of his work and he had lots of wealthy people, in addition to himself, who believed in what he was doing.

"I knew we could not be sure of what we had, but that it looked pretty damning. To stop this work with all this uncertainty was for me unacceptable. Together with Dr. Rüdiger from the Medical University of Vienna I tried to continue. So we found other money. We set out to study how DNA responds to the most modern cell phone technology, which allows a much more efficient transfer of data in a much shorter time."

Adlkofer's group did not study living rodents in comfy chambers, as did the Swedish neurosurgeon Leif Salford, described in an earlier chapter. Instead they looked carefully into a number of different human cells grown in small lab dishes and examined what happened to them after exposures quite like those that most of us get from using the phone. They examined adult cells and those from children.

The human cells that Adlkofer probed after such exposure also looked unhealthy.

"We found a ten times higher rate of broken DNA with the new 3G phones (using what is termed the UMTS system) as compared to 2G (using the older GSM system). This could be a catastrophe for the industry. It took us two years, but we finally published our work showing major damage to genetic material in cell-phone exposed human cells in the International Archives of Occupational and Environmental Health, 2008."

In the years leading up to this publication, every time Adlkofer presented a paper on the topic to meetings of the Bioelectromagnetics Society in Europe, the United States, or Asia, industry-sponsored experts came well prepared to challenge the work. Scientists working for the U.S. military and NATO — groups that used radio frequency both to communicate and to make novel weapons — went on the attack. Broken DNA does not sound like a good thing even to those not steeped in biology. After all, the destruction of DNA means that our cells have lost their ability to repair themselves, to stay under control, and eventually to suppress uncontrolled growth that is the hallmark of cancer.

Perhaps Adlkofer had figured that the complexity and elegance of the study his group had carried out would insulate it. Maybe he even thought he had acquired immunity against attack because of his many years working with industry. Or perhaps he figured that the fact that several others were repeating his study and finding the same results meant it would be accepted. On all accounts he could not have been more wrong.

By 2008, the work Adlkofer and his team at the University of Vienna had been carrying out for more than a decade suddenly made headlines in all major science journals in precisely the way a scientist never welcomes.

"Vienna Studies Withdrawn. Fraud Admitted in DNA Damage Studies in Vienna." *Science* magazine claimed that

> *. . . the only two peer-reviewed scientific papers showing that electromagneticfields (EMFs) from cell phones can cause DNA breakage are at the center of a misconduct controversy at the Medical University of Vienna (MUV). Critics had argued that the data looked too good to be real, and in May a university investigation agreed, concluding that data in both studies had been fabricated and that the papers should be retracted.*
>
> *The technician who worked on the studies [Elisabeth Kratochvil] has resigned, and the senior author on both papers [Hugo Rüdiger] initially agreed with the rector of the university to retract them. But since then, the case has become murkier as the senior author has changed his mind, saying that the technician denies wrongdoing.*

Microwave News pointed out that Science magazine got it wrong. The Viennese researchers were not lone rangers producing studies unlike everyone else. There were not just two studies showing DNA damage from radio frequency radiation, but eleven others. Despite this error, the Science magazine story was reported around the world. "Scandal Rocks Vienna Research," "Cell Phones Do Not Damage DNA."

Industry saw these headlines as a tremendous break. These scientists claiming that cell phones could be harmful had been wrong and had committed fraud — what could be clearer?

A letter to the editor by the Australian neurosurgeon Vini Khurana noted that the Science story was in fact wide of the mark. The REFLEX studies were not an isolated finding. More than a dozen different studies from highly respected researchers showed that radio frequency signals could damage DNA, alter the ability of cells to repair themselves, or cause them to die off at unusual rates. But by then the genie was out of the bottle. In a world where headlines may be all that many ever read, even if they are proved wrong eventually, the damage was done.

A Devil in Hell?

In the rush of folks arriving at the InterCity Premium Hotel in Porto Alegre a few hundred meters from the great glass modern buildings of the Health Ministry, where we met in the spring of 2009, Adlkofer kept to himself. He stood with his large head tilted down just a bit more than seemed right, even for someone who spends too much time looking down a microscope. He was dressed more elegantly than other scientists, with rimless glasses and a tailored Egyptian cotton blue shirt. Something was on his mind.

It had been about two years since Adlkofer had seen the headlines about fraud in his lab. He was still recovering, recounting, and seeking to restore himself. People who have been traumatized often talk about what happened over and over again. Adlkofer spoke about how he felt when he first learned he had been charged with fraud.

"I was just entering the boat. At this instant, my cell phone rang. I will never forget this moment ever in my life. My colleague, Professor Hugo Rüdiger, head of occupational health at the Medical University of Vienna, was on the line. 'Please, Franz, sit down.'

"This was very strange to get any call at all at this time. Rüdiger himself was in Turkey, also on holiday. When I heard his voice on the phone ordering me to get a seat, I thought someone must have died.

Rüdiger went on, 'Elisabeth has forged our data. I just got a phone call from a colleague in Vienna that she admitted that she had done this.'

"For a moment my brain froze. I had no words of reply. He was telling me that the best technician I had ever worked with, on whom our entire work rested, had done us in. Then, I blurted out, 'What are you telling me! Could this possibly be true?'

"Rüdiger replied, 'I am very sorry to tell you this, but my colleague told me that Elisabeth confessed to him. She had forged the reports.'"

Adlkofer looked uncomfortable; beads of sweat broke out on his forehead. He continued, "Frankly, I did not know what to think. I had a hard time believing my own ears. But this was a most serious matter. The future of all of our research on radio frequency signals and brain cells was at risk. My reputation would be ruined."

Adlkofer had himself mastered techniques for separating out the amino acids and other essential compounds from the proteins that keep us alive. As a teacher he had mentored dozens of younger faculty members. This role has a great tradition in Germany; there is a term for a postdoctoral mentor: *Doktorvater*, meaning roughly "doctor father" — a man who holds total dominion over his student children. He now found himself torn between loyalty to his junior lab technician and dread of the awful consequences of her alleged actions.

Back in Germany, Adlkofer tried to contact Elisabeth but failed. She had left the university and was looking for another job. He had no reason to doubt what he had been told about Elisabeth, no matter how hard it was to accept that his lab results had been fraudulent.

Adlkofer noticed the University of Vienna moved fast in attempting to control the damage to its public profile.

"The university quickly issued a press release that the data we had published showing that low levels of radio frequency signals from commonly used phones could damage DNA would have to be withdrawn from the journals *Mutation Research* and in the *International Archives of Occupational and Environmental Health*."

Once a scientist is charged with fraud, that's it — but maybe not this time. Adlkofer had two things going for him that most scientists do not. He had a lot of money from all those years working for tobacco, and he had the respect of the scientists with whom he had worked on radio frequency. He spent the next two years learning what had gone on and fighting for the record to be corrected.

Adlkofer had arrived at the conference in Brazil, where he told me his story uncertain of what lay ahead, of what this all would finally mean for someone nearing retirement. It was spring, but wind and rain can be very brisk in May there, where the weather blows straight from the Antarctic. Porto Alegre in southern Brazil was cold that week. All of us had flown through the night — there is no other way to reach this place. I'd traveled there along with Adlkofer and some two dozen other scientists to discuss the latest scientific findings on cell phones and other forms of nonionizing radiation. Porto Alegre is surrounded by some stands of original forest and assorted sprawling industrial complexes. With fewer than two million people, the area is one of the most beautiful and accessible wild regions in the country.

As we waited for the rains to abate, Adlkofer tried to tell his story from beginning to end. I had become part of his agenda, in a way that I was not fully comfortable with. Truth in science, as in much of life, depends on where you stand and who has brought you there. We were all guests of the Brazilian government at this conference convened by the International Commission for Electromagnetic Safety — a group of scientists who have been holding meetings around the world for more than a decade, seeking to promote research and policy changes. Adlkofer and I were relatively recent members.

Adlkofer had long enjoyed close contacts with many industry scientists and was astounded by what had ensued when his group began to produce results the cell phone industry did not like.

"I'd been conducting research on the fundamental and basic science of cell phones for three decades. As we set up the studies of radio frequency signals, of course, I relied on industry help to do so. Industry scientists had been my close colleagues throughout. They were not at all happy with this work that we had published in Mutation Research, in 2005. They let me know it. This study belonged to the REFLEX project, which had received nearly three million euros from the European Union and was well funded by my own foundation, the Radiation and Nuclear Safety Authority (STUK) of Finland and the Swiss government. No direct industry money was involved.

"We found that radio frequency, especially at the level then found in regular cell phones using GSM radiation, caused big and obvious toxic effects in human fibroblasts.

We exposed fibroblasts from persons young and old to electromagnetic fields used to modulate the carrier frequencies of mobile phone radiation. Fibroblasts from younger persons have a slower increase in DNA strand breaks and a faster decrease; this means their repair systems were obviously better. Several hundred pages of our work also appeared in a special issue under the Verum Foundation final report of the REFLEX project.

"Different groups were involved with different ways of charting cell damage. We looked at gene expression. We counted and measured rates of cell growth and death. We examined how the immune system responded. The most important results showed genotoxic impacts. We presented the data several times, including at Bioelectromagnetics Society meetings. Each time efforts were made to explain why we were wrong. So we refined our studies and got the same results. They knew what was coming was not to their liking."

Having worked with Elisabeth for nearly a decade, Adlkofer could not believe that she would have betrayed their work so easily.

"I can't prove this, but here's what I think they did. The industry never liked this work. From the first they heard about it, they set out to discredit it. I had seen this happen with tobacco science so often, especially at the hands of the American companies. Yet suddenly it was happening to me. They hired people to show that our results could not be replicated. But these groups carried out their studies in a way that our data could not be reproduced. So what happened next?

"Today, this same Professor Lerchl — whom industry supported to attack our work — is the chairman of the independent government commission for the science on nonionizing radiation. He has written a book that he published himself, outlining his story in this sorry episode. He claims to have determined the truth, when what he really did was to shanghai and undermine our work. This is a man who wouldn't know the truth if it fell on him!" What happened next dumbfounded Adlkofer. Before the ink was dry on the declarations of guilt made by those appointed to succeed him, and before any final decision had been reached about the accusation of fraud, the rector of the university ordered the laboratory to have all records of this research destroyed, completely wiped out.

"I refused. I knew something few others could. During the time that my technician was allegedly cooking the books, there was no way she could have possibly known how to do so. Nobody in our labs, not even me, had the information on the codes. The codes were not known to any of us. Nobody.

"As I was struggling with all this, then something even more strange happened. The ethics committee set up by the rector confirmed that the data should be considered forged. And they reached this conclusion without ever trying to talk with me directly. I soon found out that something was fishy. I got a phone call tipping me off. It turned out that the chairman of this foundation's ethics committee — the very same Professor Lerchl who had raised such a fuss about our work and demanded that we retract it — was himself directly sponsored by the telecommunications industry and his university received millions from them as well."

The battle began in earnest.

"We fought hard. We did not accept any claim to destroy the data. We made use of this conflict-of-interest information in talking to the journals. We demanded that the university set up a new ethics committee with a chair not from the industry.

"The rector finally agreed. He set up an ethics committee with a new chairman, while two of its three members remained in their positions. This means that a conflict of interest could not be fully excluded.

"After some investigation, I was told that this new committee would reach the same conclusion that the data had been fabricated. I wrote to them that before I could accept this, I would like to read the protocol of the ethics committee.

"They refused to send it to me. So I went to Vienna with Hugo Rüdiger and we went through the report. At the end, I said, 'I do not see any proof that the data has been fabricated.'

"The rector's representative tried to convince me that I should read between the lines.

"But by then, Rüdiger and I had managed to speak with Elisabeth. She had been avoiding us for months. I didn't know if she was ill or merely heartsick. When we finally spoke, I learned that she had never confessed to forgery at all. She had been set up. When she was finally asked directly about this, Elisabeth said she hadn't done it. The whole story of fraud was itself a fraud!"

Was it really possible that a major university would go through an investigation on such a flimsy pretext? Elisabeth's story gets harder to confirm beyond that point, but according to Adlkofer, she was adamant. She never admitted fudging the radio frequency radiation data.

149

The journals in which Adlkofer's REFLEX team's work first appeared, *Mutation Research* and the *Archives of Occupational and Environmental Health,* investigated on their own. They determined that the Adlkofer lab reports should not be retracted and that their reports were valid. They agreed that cell phone microwave-like signals like those in our phones today can profoundly alter the ability of cells to repair themselves. The peer-reviewed science is there. Since this extraordinary review took place, several other investigators in other countries have produced the same results — cell phone radiation does damage DNA.

The REFLEX team's extensive research program on the biological effects of cell phone radiation found harmful effects. Its leader was accused of fraud. Then he was totally exonerated.

How has the story been told so far? Aside from a few trade journals, no major newspapers have reported the fact that the so-called fraud of Vienna — publicized at one point around the world — is not actually a fraud at all. Der Spiegel, Germany's highest circulation newsweekly, was sarcastic at the time. Imagine, they joked, the professors think cell phones could be dangerous. In 2008, the magazine ran a Photoshopped image of Professor Rüdiger. It showed him sitting next to an attractive young girl on a cell phone. The notation called him Professor Unrat. In Heinrich Mann's novel of the same name, Unrat loses his dignity when he becomes obsessed with Lola — a cabaret singer. Marlene Dietrich became famous for hypnotically chanting the song "Falling in Love Again" in the film version of the book, *The Blue Angel.*

"The best journalists are with Der Spiegel and I thought they had understood what had happened and would report the truth. They did not," says Adlkofer.

Adlkofer and Rüdiger are nearing the end of their work, but Adlkofer is not stopping at this point. He refuses to accept retirement as an out and is working to ensure that the results stand. He proudly notes that several recent papers confirm that pulsed digital radio frequency radiation can damage DNA. When asked why most studies on the question have been negative, he retorts, "Follow the money."

What of the younger researchers who have been close observers or involved in this drama? Many of them are afraid. Some are even publishing under pseudonyms to avoid being targeted. Perhaps they've learned to be very careful. Being careful is the hallmark of a good scientist. So, it seems, is being quiet.

As I left Porto Alegre and caught my plane back to North America, I reflected on the fact that about a hundred million people in Brazil use cell phones today and many of them are under age twenty. Many cities there restrict the placement of radio towers, keeping them far from schools and bedroom windows — something that many, more developed, nations have not attempted.

The impact of Adlkofer's work showing genetic damage from cell phone exposures — a finding that has a long but little-known history — is hard to overestimate. This was not the effort of a lone scientist working in a garage, but the result of teams of scientists using the same methods, repeating the same work, in different laboratories. And the findings confirmed results produced decades earlier by several other teams of investigators. Here was a group of distinguished researchers showing what many physicists assumed was impossible. Damage occurred to cells that had nothing at all to do with detectible changes in heat. Radio frequency signals at levels that could be found every day caused havoc inside cells, blocking their ability to function normally and breaking down the brain's barrier to pollutants or drugs in the bloodstream.

In their investigations, Adlkofer's team found that the newly launched 3G phones were much worse than the now outdated 2G phones.

A hundred million cell phone users in Brazil.

Five billion around the world.

A global public health problem is getting worse.

7

THE TROUBLE WITH MEN

The world is not dangerous because of those who do harm but because of those who look at it without doing anything.
~Albert Einstein

Eric and Nancy, both in their mid-thirties, began sensing that biological clock that says it's now or never. In 2007, they got married, bought a home, and tried to start a family. Successful computer programmers, they had plunked down several hundred dollars for high tech gear that measured the tiny surge in hormones that signaled precisely when one of the three hundred thousand eggs from Nancy's ovaries moved into the end of one of the fallopian tubes, where it could be fertilized. After two years, it was starting to look like now had become never. They had tried everything that doctors and well-intentioned family members had suggested. Red blankets, vitamin E, long walks, deep talks, and diligent coupling had not produced pregnancy. Every morning, Nancy took her temperature and tested her urine. When she registered a bit warmer than usual with a spurt in hormones, Nancy would call Eric, who had often left for work before dawn

153

and always kept his cell phone in his front pocket. He talked on his phone more than five thousand minutes a month. Eric would dash home to make sure that they were able to give it their best shot. Lovemaking had become work. They were beginning to feel like failures.

Libby still doesn't know why she could not get pregnant forty years ago. But she has long had her suspicions. She and her young husband, John, had grown up knowing each other slightly, but after attending the same college, they fell in love and got married when they were just twenty-one. Their fathers had shared offices at the largest municipal energy utility in America — the L.A. Department of Water and Power. When their wives were both pregnant, the dads laid bets on which one of their children would be born first. After John's birth, Libby followed two weeks later.

On vacation trips with their electrical engineer dad, Libby and her siblings visited power plants, substations, electricity generating dams, turbines, and generators. Their skin would tingle and their hair would stand on end because of the high-voltage electricity surging around them. At family gatherings after Libby and John got married, their parents would toast to the grandchildren they hoped for. Libby and John were eager to start a family. As months and years passed without pregnancy, they went through prolonged heartbreak.

Libby's dad, Floyd L. Goss, a Berkeley graduate in electrical engineering, worked for years overseeing electrical line installations in California, the fastest growing state in the nation. Libby's mom later wondered if what she believed was a dream job setting up high-power electricity might have caused the array of chronic health ailments that her husband developed by his early forties.

Nobody then thought to ask whether Libby and John's infertility could have anything to do with their unusual childhood vacations or where their fathers had worked.

"My mother used to say that when my dad was living in the desert looking after the huge number of high-power transmission lines they were building then, his eyes were totally whited out. She didn't know whether it was from the desert or from the electrical exposures. He always wore sunglasses even back then and had such pale pale blue eyes, but after those trips his eyes looked almost alien."

After years of not being able to conceive, and painful recriminations, Libby and John parted.

Eric and Nancy were more fortunate. Of the many experts they consulted about what was beginning to look like infertility, one suggested that they try something radical. Keep their cell phones completely off of their bodies and use them only for texting or with a corded headset for two months. Then try again, while limiting their tinkering with computers. While this seemed a bit oddball, they decided it would not be that hard to make this effort. Nothing else had worked.

Within a year, they became parents. Of course, this could simply be a coincidence. Nevertheless, a growing number of scientific reports — in rodents, insects, and real people — are finding that cell phone radiation can interfere with this most exquisitely sensitive part of human life — our ability to become parents when we choose to do so.

Love might make the world go around, but small amounts of electric current hold our cells together and keep us alive and well. Our bodies contain billions of brilliantly organized microscopic cells made up of many different types of molecules that protect us and keep us alive. With a precision that convinces some of us of holy intentions, proteins are triggered to govern growth and repair damage, and specially designed cells are organized to fend off infection. Each molecule within our body consists of atoms held together by chemical bonds. A single misstep and the whole thing can fall apart. Every single atom contains a nucleus, neutrons, protons, and electrons — basic elements of all matter. Electrons circle atoms in our bodies, determining when, whether, and with what materials they may combine.

Balanced charges are stable and hard to disturb. Unpaired or free electrons can be dangerous and very unsteady and constantly seek to hook up with other biological tissues by stealing electrons with which to bond.

Atoms have mostly stable bonds because their outer electron orbiting shells are packed with neatly paired electrons. Free radicals are the cougars of the atomic world, crafty, stealthy, always seeking out the weakest electrons with which they can align just long enough to weaken the strong, neat atomic bond, and move on. At their best, the unfettered electrons of free radicals can break through and blow up invasive viruses and bacteria before they manage to multiply and cause prolonged illness or death. At their worst, unchained radicals can roam about destroying healthy parts of the body, creating smooth sailing for opportunistic infections or worse. Smokers have more wrinkles, less resilient lungs, and more chronic bronchitis because they take in more damaging agents from the extensive array of unbound radicals found in tobacco smoke. People who regularly incur exposures to chemical pollutants and those who have the good fortune to live long lives also show signs of free-radical damage.

If we are lucky, we don't inherit defective genes from our parents and we don't live and work in environments that place damaging chemicals within our bodies. If we are very lucky, we also manage to eat the right foods at the right times. And if we are even more lucky, our bodies organize ways to neutralize free radicals that occur simply because we are exposed to sunlight and oxygen and other compounds that naturally release un-bonded electrons. Well-defended with good nutrition, exercise, and/or good genes, we can neutralize rampaging free radicals, absorb the hits, and move on. Those of us who are of grandparent age or beyond grew up in a world free from microwaves, which surround our children and grandchildren today. Whatever damaging free radicals we encountered as children were mostly tied with early industrializing chemicals or radiation — exposures to agents like asbestos, benzene, and pesticides are now many times lower than in the past.

Chemicals can smell bad. High doses of X-rays can burn the skin and cause the hair to fall out. In contrast, microwave frequencies of the sort produced by modern cell phones remain below the capacity of most humans to perceive them. How can we understand whether this silent, odorless form of exposure does anything at all to our health? Why should we think that this is even a possibility? After all, our bodies require tiny amounts of electricity to keep our hearts beating, our blood flowing, and brains in control.

Despite their invisible and noiseless nature, radio frequencies have much in common with some of the chemical hazards that give rise to environmental protection around the world today. Radio frequencies have the capacity to unleash precisely the same sort of free radicals and to disrupt the invisible cellular bonds that hold molecules together. Certain sizes of radio frequencies also can send too many of the wrong type of heat-shock proteins that normally fix damage within cells, protect our brains from taking in harmful agents, and generally keep our DNA working to defend our bodies. When it comes to heat-shock proteins, Mae West got it wrong — too much of a good thing is not always better.

Radio frequency signals of the sort emitted by cell phones resonate with our bodies and can release insidious free radicals into the bloodstream, where they end up moving around to places they shouldn't reach. The very existence of free radicals within the body causes the force with which blood moves within the arteries to rise, effectively increasing one's blood pressure. When we are attacked or in danger for a short period of time, higher blood pressure can be a good thing, speeding up the heart, allowing us to run faster, and move and think more quickly, although not necessarily improving our efficiency or precision. But for any longer period, sustained higher blood pressure strains the rest of the body, weakens blood vessels, arteries, and veins, and increases the chance that the heart or brain will be overwhelmed by surges in force or broken clots of blood that can cut off oxygen, killing muscles and ultimately ending life. Even if they do not noticeably raise blood pressure, one of the consequences of having an abundance of free radicals coursing around the body is that they open up something that is best left shut. They weaken the capacity of the brain to protect us from foreign materials

Young, Powerful Men

Young men in powerful jobs tend to dress casually today. Hand-rolled neckties, gold cufflinks, and hand-tailored suits have given way to peacoats, corduroys, limited edition T-shirts, designer work shirts and pants, and cordovans. But self-confident gentlemen have found other ways to signal status by what they wear. The number and types of wireless devices clipped to their belts or stored in their pockets, or around their arms or wrists, indicate how important someone else thinks they are and how much money they have to spend. Everyone understands that pregnant women should be kept free from dangers, both physical and chemical. But not so many appreciate that the chemical and physical environments a man moves through in the four months before his sperm impregnates the egg or eggs of his partner — or even whether the sperm reaches an egg at all — affects the chance of producing healthy children. It is not disputed that alcoholics and drug addicts tend to have sickly offspring, if they have any. But few have heard that studies in many nations find that men who keep cell phones turned on in their pockets for hours a day have fewer sperm with more deformities. The eighteenth-century French philosopher Diderot explained that a central difference between men and women lies with how their bodies house their primary sex organs. For women,

the ovaries, of course, are protected inside, while for men there is simply less protection. Remember those sailors who used radar to avoid
making babies on shore leave? They instinctively knew they could
disrupt their ability to reproduce. The so-called testicular barrier —
the delicate skin covering the scrotum — is not really a barrier at all.
The membrane covering the testes is about one hundred times more
sensitive to chemical exposures than any other skin surface.

It doesn't matter how much of a tough guy you are.

During the first few months of prenatal life, cells start to form that
eventually become sperm-producing organs in the adult — the sem-
iniferous tubules. Sertoli cells are basically the boy-making factories
within these tubules that release male hormones at the right time and
place to start the process that leads to the production of millions of
sperm. At adolescence, these cells start to mature along with the testes.

Sperm are among the fastest and speediest-growing cells in the
body. They must travel heroic distances to succeed in fertilizing an
egg. As one of half a billion swimming cells in ejaculate, a single
sperm leaves the body at a speed that is faster than most humans can
run — about ten miles an hour. One old joke holds that the reason it
takes so many sperm to fertilize a single egg is that the sperm don't
know how to ask for directions. Indeed, some sperm lose direction,
some lose energy, and all die in a few days. The healthier all sperm
are, the better the chance that a single one will succeed. Sperm have
a head and a tail that propels them forward. They can be examined
and scored in terms of how well they swim, their shape, and their
speed. For their short existence, sperm have only one job — to swim
upstream to win the prize of entry into a large healthy egg. The egg
doesn't just lie there, it busily sends out chemicals that attract and
draw the sperm through its tough membrane, providing that other
things have not impeded the process. Sperm that swim fastest and
straightest have the best chance of success and tend to be those with

the longest, strongest tails to whip them along. If a sperm were the size of a human, a successful one would need to stay on course and swim from Los Angeles to Hawaii to arrive at its target.

When it comes to investigating whether cell phones impact the exquisite process of human reproduction, we are in the midst of yet another vast uncontrolled experiment on ourselves. Almost all young adult men and women are using cell phones around the world today. In the United States more teenagers are using cell phones than in most other countries of the world. The Kaiser Family Foundation reported that some American teenagers spend as much as eighteen hours a day engaging with computers, electronics, and various mobile devices, and the average teen uses various gadgets about seven hours a day. At its most elegant and straight-forward execution, as in the study of pharmaceutical agents, medical science works best by comparing those with exposures to those without, commonly called the control group. When evaluating drugs, we can expose some people and leave others unexposed. We can be sure that whatever difference occurs is due to the differences in drugs used. But with cell phones being used by nearly all young adults today, where can we find the unexposed control group? Besides, unlike toxic chemical exposure, our lives depend on small amounts of electric impulses. So figuring out the marginal impact of added electromagnetic radiation on our health is not merely a matter of coming up with the traditional dose and response, but requires an entirely new approach

Is That a Free Radical in Your Pocket?

Researchers at the famed Cleveland Clinic produced some fascinating analyses of how sperm are affected by cell phone radiation. A report from researchers at the clinic in 2008 garnered headlines around the world, such as "Cell Phones Lower Sperm Count." Like many findings in medicine, this work came about from an incidental observation by an astute scientist. Often men who could afford to seek help from the Cleveland Clinic would show up clad in Vittorio Russo or Kenneth Cole loafers, designer blue jeans, with a sleek BlackBerry, and maybe another cell phone or pager as well, clipped onto their leather belts. In the summer, they kept these phones in their pants pockets.

Ashok Agarwal trained at Harvard and is one of the world's foremost experts in what is called andrology — the study of what makes males male, the biology of the male reproductive system. Currently director of the Andrology Laboratory and Reproductive Tissue Bank at the clinic, Agarwal has written more than four hundred peer-reviewed articles. A simple questionnaire Agarwal handed out came up with what appeared to be a stunning breakthrough: Men with the lowest sperm counts were significantly more likely to keep their phones on their bodies all the time, usually in their pockets. By all these measures, men who used no cell phones had far more healthy sperm than those who used a phone two or four or more hours a day, and those who reported using a phone for four hours or more had the lowest and sickliest sperm counts of all. Remarkably, out of 364 men in the clinic, more than half were on their phones for two hours a day. Only 10 percent reported not using a phone much at all.

Agarwal's team devised a very clever tactic. Each person became his own control. Sperm samples from thirty-four individual clinic volunteers were taken into the laboratory and split into two parts — one part received no exposure to radio frequency, while the other was exposed for one hour to levels of radiation from a cell phone held about an inch away from the test tube — to approximate the distance between the testes and a man's pocket. Sperm exposed to the highest levels of cell phone radiation had the most deformities and the worst swimming abilities.

The Cleveland researchers referred to their results, in the customary voice of science, as "preliminary," and duly called for more research. The fact is, more research is always called for. It is the one thing on which all scientists agree. Agarwal, at least in public, seems to be awkwardly hedging his bets. He told *Newsweek* in 2009 that he keeps his cell phone turned off and in his pants pocket, because "I already have two children." Despite what must have been a glib retort, no one could seriously propose using cell phones as a form of birth control.

Gumming Up the Engines of Evolution

Agarwal is not the only researcher to show that radio frequency signals affect the amount and health of sperm. The Cleveland Clinic findings are not quite as preliminary as the researchers may have thought, nor are they solitary. Since the turn of this century, there have been independent scientific reports from other distinguished researchers in seven different countries — Australia, Japan, Hungary, Poland, Turkey, China, and the United States — showing that cell phone radiation seriously impairs the sperm of both mice and men. In 2010, Cambridge University–trained, award-winning Laureate Professor John Aitken reported on a parallel series of projects that also studied test tube cultures of human sperm exposed to radio frequency radiation at levels that can be produced by cell phones. His nationally funded Australian Research Council Center of Excellence in Biotechnology and Development states as its mission, "the analysis of the specification and differentiation of male germ cells." The group is devoted to one thing: understanding all the factors that can affect men's ability to become fathers if and when they choose to do so.

Aitken's center has shown that after little more than a day of exposure to cell phone radiation, sperm become sluggish swimmers. The Australian team used three different levels of cell phone radiation and found that the highest exposures produced the weakest sperm with the most damage. This finding shows what is called a dose-response relationship: As the dose goes up, so does the damage. Wherever such a connection can be made between a given exposure and a given response, it strengthens the grounds for thinking that there is a direct association.

Intrigued by these findings, Aitken's researchers have developed a theory of what could be going on. They know that cell phone radiation does not directly damage the sperm's DNA straight on, as happens when X-rays hit. Rather, they believe that cell phone radiation weakens the ability of a sperm cell to get sufficient oomph needed for its marathon swim from the testes to the place securely inside the female where it can impregnate the egg. Energy for all this movement comes from thousands of furnacelike mitochondrial cells in sperm that work as a kind of onboard engine. If electrons that hold together these cellular machines fall out of place after exposure to cell phone radiation, this produces dangerous free radicals. These rogue materials carom about, seeking whatever alliance they can, and rob sperm of their vigor. If enough free radicals are generated through leaking mitochondria, this can actually harm DNA by weakening the basic structure of genetic material. Think of a rubber band. You can snap it many times, but at some point it will break. Free radicals can stretch the bands that hold cells together, eventually snapping them entirely. Studies on the capacity of radio frequency signals to impair sperm are mounting, as more researchers at infertility clinics around the world have begun to ask about cell phone use. Hungarian analysts from that nation's top-ranked medical school at the University of Szeged found that men who used cell phones the most had the slowest and worst-swimming sperm. In 2007, a team of Polish investigators from an infertility clinic at the medical center in Lublin released similar results — men reporting the highest use of cell phones had the lowest and sickest sperm. In 2006, researchers from the Gulhane Military Medical Academy in Etlik, Ankara, Turkey, showed significantly impaired movement in human sperm exposed to cell-phone-type radiation in studies quite like those in Cleveland and Australia.

So many different things can affect sperm that it's tempting to believe that radio frequency signals are not really playing any role at all. Perhaps these men who use cell phones heavily also tend to drink more alcohol or work in more dangerous jobs? In fact, in carrying out these studies researchers have done as much as they can to rule out these other factors. Still the results remain — something about RF is causing sperm to lose their way, become sickly, and die. A recent well-designed experiment from a group in Melaka Manipal Medical College in India is especially worrisome. If their work is correct, the way boys today use cell phones will make it less likely they can become fathers later in life. These researchers started with young white rats about three months old — comparable to teenage boys in development — and exposed them for just one hour a day to radiation from a smart phone — one operating, like most phones today, at between 900 and 1,800 megahertz — placed just under the rat's cage. Just to be sure that the mere physical presence of the phone itself was not causing something weird to happen, they also placed a phone without a battery under the cage of another group of rats. They found that cell phone exposure did not change the temperature of the head of the rat, so it did not produce any heat. But the rats exposed to the actual cell phone signals developed significantly more damaging free radicals in their blood, reduced sperm counts, and lowered amounts of male hormones.

Other studies from Athens led by Lukas Margaritis, one of Greece's leading researchers on electromagnetic radiation, working with Adamantia Fragopoulou, is also troubling. Using the well-studied fruit fly *Drosophila*, they have come up with evidence that cell phone radiation can kill cells located in the reproductive organs of this lowly, prolific little fly. With remarkable patience, steady hands, and magnifying microscopes, they have painstakingly dissected the ovaries and testes of these tiny flies. Just six minutes a day of exposure to cell phone radiation from real phones throws a crowbar into these minute and vital organs.

Preliminary?

What do all of these studies tell us at this point? Men are not mice, to be sure. But we match them in deep, consequential ways, as the human and rodent genome projects have confirmed. Genetic evolution tells us that humans share more genes with rodents than with dogs or chickens. From the remarkable number of common silent mutations that we share, we now know that at one point long before science was a possibility, about eighty-five million years ago, rodents and humans had a common ancestor.

All this work teasing out the various mechanisms involved in derailing and deforming millions of sperm and throwing animals off track and out of sorts, unraveling the myriad ways that radio frequency signals affect our cells, is worthy of a Nobel Prize or three. Whether it will garner that level of public recognition remains to be seen. But the number of scientists convinced of the value of this approach and the importance of these findings is growing. Scientists are devising automated ways to picture the full range of biological impacts of cell phone signals on living things.

Scientists other than Franz Adlkofer are looking at DNA. Some are taking the whole enterprise a step further and looking directly into the core of sperm and brain cells, into the very structure and function of genetic material in DNA. Whether taken from the head of human sperm or the cells of the rat brain, evidence is accumulating that radio frequency radiation can make DNA spiral out of control, leaving behind trails of broken parts.

Throughout evolution our normal DNA has been frequently damaged and fixed. That's why we survive the daily assaults of oxygen and sunlight and the free radicals they naturally generate. But the modern world presents biology with entirely new challenges in kind and degree. The evolution of life on earth is now changing because of the radical changes we have made to the environment. What will it take for all of these "preliminary findings" that cell phone radiation harms our fundamental biology not to be considered preliminary?

We must remember that we live in a world in which some continue to believe evolution itself is a sort of "preliminary theory."

8

CELL PHONES CURE ALZHEIMER'S!

If they can get you asking the wrong questions,
they don't have to worry about answers.
~Thomas Pynchon

The difference between life and death is solely electric. We contain the same chemicals and liquids when we are living, breathing, talking, and walking as we do in the moments right after death. When we are alive, electricity streams from and to the brain because we are made up of atoms, every single one of which contains protons, neutrons, and electrons. The comedian Dave Barry once quipped that "electricity is actually made up of extremely tiny particles called electrons that you cannot see with the naked eye unless you have been drinking." But in fact, no matter how much nor what you may have imbibed, you will never be able to see that protons have positive charges, neutrons have none, and electrons are negatively charged. For more than a century, medical researchers around the world have built methods to find and fix diseases or broken bodies, relying on our natural invisible electric properties.

While we are electric beings, our bodies and brains are not wired with miles of cabling like televisions. The circuits within our bodies connect when electricity leaps from one nerve cell to the next, creating a flow between positive and negative charges. When resting, a cell has more positively charged sodium and potassium cations that carry a positive charge right within its center or nucleus. Negatively charged chloride ions reside outside. Electrical opposites really do attract. Potassium and sodium ions sit on opposite ends of a closed gate, longing for union. To send a message, a cell opens the gate so that these attracted ions can complete a circuit. The whole effort takes place with no buzzing sensation or warmth, at speeds that we cannot detect. Even at rest, bare nerve cells pulsate imperceptibly. In fact, by the time the skin feels any change in temperature or any buzz from an electrical signal, whether on our hands or the surface of our skulls, electrical impulses have been at work far below the surface for some time. The brain, as we have learned, senses neither heat nor pain. One can imagine that our brain's lack of direct sensation provides a kind of protection against what would otherwise be unbearable suffering. Our small brains control our large bodies, sending and receiving messages of movement, directing chemical couriers to turn on and off, and staying cool as the proverbial cucumber, so long as we don't subject them to prolonged currents designed to warm tissue.

The Electric Heart

Willem Einthoven's father, a parish medical officer on the island of Java in the Dutch East Indies (now Indonesia), died of a stroke at age forty-five in 1866. Four years later, when he was ten, the fatherless Einthoven sailed back to his ancestral home in Holland with his widowed mother and five siblings. His father's sudden and early death may have served as a cautionary tale. From a young age Einthoven engaged in especially brisk and vigorous activities, convinced of the value of staying fit. By age eighteen he'd started medical training at the same university that his father had attended in Utrecht.

Thoroughly schooled in physics and eager to confirm the value of his own athletic abilities at the start of his career in medical research, Einthoven gravitated naturally to characterizing the human heart. For centuries, the steadiness of the heartbeat and the regularity of its sounds had fascinated medical experts and poets. Turning comforting thumping heart sounds into repeatable sound measures proved challenging. For more than a century scientists had understood that the body's hardest working muscle depended on tiny amounts of electricity, whether awake or asleep. A complicated experimental apparatus called a capillary electrometer used a glass tube filled with the liquid heavy metal mercury to project images of each heartbeat onto a photographic plate. One end of the tube stood immersed in diluted acid. The up-and-down movements of the mercury column were projected onto slowly moving photosensitive paper, producing images that proved difficult to decipher.

Most doctors at the beginning of the twentieth century could not imagine any practical use would come of the effort to characterize the heartbeat in a reproducible manner. Time passed by heartbeats or other markers was thought of, if at all, as one of those immutable aspects of life — gone, unrecoverable, and unremarkable. But Einthoven was convinced that it was both possible and important to mark time with heartbeats in a way that could be reproduced. He set about to create a device to record the steady stream of electrical activity in the heart that would tell physicians important things about the person in whose body any heart rested. He knew that a single beat begins when a tiny pulse of current causes the top of the heart muscle to become taut, sending blood coursing into the arteries. The idea of metering, measuring, and marking patterns of heartbeats fascinated the meticulous Einthoven. He soon turned to another device to provide a more reliable method. At the core of the cumbersome string galvanometer a silver-coated, meters-long, super-thin quartz filament lay between two powerful electromagnets. The first machines were massive, requiring a steady stream of water to keep the electromagnets from overheating, five people to run the equipment, the space of a small office, and they weighed as much as four men — some six hundred pounds. Patients had to sit motionless with both their arms and their left leg immersed in buckets of salt water that would conduct electric current from their skin to the quartz filament. As the heart beat, the quartz filament moved slightly, signaling the conduction of electric current. Images of this faint but steady movement were magnified and projected through a tiny slot onto a slowly moving photographic plate. One could see steady, regular, predictable patterns of healthy heart rhythms as well as chaotic patterns from life-threatening arrhythmias with menacingly irregular pulses.

Einthoven received the Nobel Prize in Physiology or Medicine in 1924, for this important work that led to the creation of today's mechanized electrocardiogram (ECG). In his sixties he painstakingly charted the onset and patterns of his own elevated blood pressure and its associated symptoms — blinding headaches, dizziness, and instability. Hypertension was a disease that could be named but could not be reliably treated. As he predicted in soulful letters to his daughter when he became bedridden, Einthoven did not reach the retirement age of seventy. He died when he was sixty-seven — just a few years after being awarded the Nobel.

The Electric Brain

The 1920s were an electrifying time in science and the rest of the world. Prejudice against the unnatural nature of electricity had largely subsided, cooled by the dramatic impacts of electric lighting and the telephone. Campaigns against the spread of electricity or telephone poles or pylons in England led by prominent intellectuals like John Maynard Keynes had foundered, as city homes and apartments throughout the industrial world switched from smoky, smelly gas lighting to lightbulbs. In 1924, the same year that Einthoven received the Nobel for developing the ECG to depict electrical patterns of heartbeats, the German psychiatrist and neuroscientist Hans Berger constructed the first stunning electrical portraits of regular currents within the brain. In his scientific pursuits, Berger followed Einthoven's path and began to characterize brain patterns with the finicky mercury-filled capillary electrometer, eventually moving to the steadier string galvanometer, which reliably displayed differences in the size, type, and patterns of brain waves.

With Berger's device, long-imagined electrical activity in the brain could actually be seen as striking, thin black lines projected onto a slowly moving piece of photographically sensitive paper. Berger's spectacular images of brain activity laid the foundation for the electroencephalogram (EEG) as a way to capture both normal and off-kilter patterns of the brain. Weighing only about three pounds, the brain contains about a hundred billion neurons, each one of which is either completely off in a state of rest or completely on when sending an impulse. These neurons connect to one another through up to a hundred trillion synapses or connections that are made when chemical messengers or transmitters link positive and negative charges. Electrodes applied to the scalp pick up otherwise imperceptible electrical activity produced by the simultaneous actions of neurons as they complete billions of circuits.

Just before the start of the world's Great Depression of 1929, Berger published a paper showing that longer, slower, and bigger delta waves signaled deep sleep, while faster, shorter alpha and beta waves indicated relaxed or alert conscious thoughts. Despite its breakthrough nature, Berger did not receive the Nobel for this innovative work. In one of many cruel edicts, Hitler refused to allow any Jewish scientist to accept such a prize in 1936. Berger's invention had opened up an exciting new frontier in understanding the electrical nature of the brain, but couldn't spare his mind from the ravages of depression induced by the rise of Nazism and the menacing political world in which he lived. Berger lost his eligibility for the prize when he took his own life in 1941.

The role of electricity in consciousness itself was one of the many topics that Robert O. Becker pursued as a trailblazing physician researcher studying the body, brain, and heart electric in the mid-twentieth century. Studying the lowly salamander, physician researcher Becker showed that electric stimulation could either induce or disturb brain waves during deep sleep. Salamanders that had been anesthetized chemically displayed the same deep, slow delta brain waves as those that slept soundly. Becker went on to ask whether the change in the brain's electrical activity was the cause or the consequence of the animal's apparent anesthesia. When a minute current passed through the head of a salamander, the animal lay immobile, unresponsive to pain, and basically unconscious. Using a much more sophisticated type of EEG, Becker soon had his answer: Small amounts of electric current could indeed create the same deep state of loss of sensation and pain relief as chemical anesthetics.

The Electric Doctor

Trained as an orthopedic surgeon, Becker was a scientist's scientist who had started his research career fascinated with the fact that salamanders that had their legs severed could grow new ones. His first thought upon seeing this happen was that this had to be some sort of fluke. However, a set of experiments showed that minute inherent electric currents set the stage for a remarkable process of regrowth. Becker published articles on the role of electric current in this astonishing phenomenon in the top-ranking journals *Science* and *Nature*. His research not only established that regrowth happened, but that natural electric currents directly built the new limbs by eliciting the formation of vital new bone and tissue. He also demonstrated that tiny amounts of external current applied at critical stages of growth could either accelerate or interfere with the process of regeneration.

In the popular book *The Body Electric*, published in 1985, Becker explained that many physicians saw broken bones as nothing but a problem of carpentry, requiring a few screws, plates, or nails. His work showed that this was a complete misunderstanding of the complexity of the skeleton. When the first true fishes of the Devonian period developed some four hundred million years ago with skeletons inside their bodies, this provided a fundamental advance in evolution. Within the body, bone is alive and provides an efficient protective matrix for muscles and tendons and for valuable internal organs, such as the brain.

> *Bone is extraordinary in structure, too. It's stronger than cast iron in resisting compression but, if killed by X rays or by cutting off its blood supply (barely adequate to start with), it collapses into mush.* (The Body Electric, 1985, p. 119)

The idea of limb regeneration can seem like science fiction. Nevertheless, Becker knew that a salamander, an amphibian with a backbone, just one step lower than the frog, could regrow its tail, legs, eyes, ears, and up to a third of its brain and half of its heart. He also had come across several hundred cases of children who regrew their fingertips after various childhood accidents. Becker was able to show that this natural regrowth took place as long as their severed digits were kept clean and were allowed to develop without medical intervention.

Becker was puzzled by what seemed miraculous evidence of regrowth across species. As an orthopedic surgeon he reasoned that bones actually do not heal from within. Instead, fractured bones recruit new tissue by turning on the formation of bone from the bone marrow and the periosteum, the bone's fibrous covering. Becker was able to show that any healed fracture comes about from the generation of fresh bone that grows over the break, forming a kind of homegrown splint that places newly made support on top of old splintered pieces. In a way the healthy healing of fractures should be thought of as a type of regeneration that proceeds through complex but predictable stages. After the initial break, first a blood clot forms that provides the basis for a seed bud, called a blastema, on which new bone can start to form. This in turn allows the production of a bony nugget or callus, which provides the milieu upon which new bone can then be laid down. What starts out as relatively soft, bloody, spongy material ends up becoming hardened bone through a process termed ossification. Becker conducted a number of innovative studies that proved that in the course of bone healing and regrowth, whether in the salamander or in humans with hard-to-heal fractures, natural electric current provides the critical component. As an orthopedist, Becker saw a number of patients whose broken legs simply would not heal. In these cases, a person faces the prospect of crippling immobility and lifelong pain. A young man who had sustained a bone crushing accident while farming had continued to work with his unhealed stump of a foot wrapped in bandages covered by rubber work boots. The area had become badly infected and Becker had no idea whether he could help. First he cleaned off or debrided all compromised tissue. Then he applied sterile salt solution. The hardworking fellow agreed to rest in bed as a contraption delivered a small amount of electric current to the wet area via a small silver blanket. Within a few days, all signs of infection were gone. Within two weeks, for the first time in more than a year, the young man could stand on his wounded leg. Becker had reasoned that applying a slight bit of direct electric current similar to that which occurs in successful spontaneous healing would prompt the process of regrowth that had failed to occur naturally. In fact, in this and several other cases, his hunch proved correct. Electromagnetic radiation directly applied to these failed breaks accelerated the repair of bone and tissue.

Diathermy — literally "through heat" — was a medical technology considered a basic tool of physical therapy for many years. Stiff muscles can respond nicely to microwaves that warm deep tissues, enhance movement, and drain inflammations. First devised in Berlin in 1907, by the 1930s diathermy was broadly used for many applications, although every so often someone would complain of bad skin burns from prolonged use. This therapeutic use of microwave radiation in medicine involved the careful application of certain wavelengths to tender muscles and bones — a subject of great interest to those of us now afflicted with what used to be thought of as the inevitable creakiness of advancing years.

Today the uses of various types of current in medicine are extensive. Some of these involve relatively high amounts of direct current to kill cells or reset an irregular heartbeat, but other applications rely on tiny levels of electricity to promote growth of bone and skin. One of the most widely used applications of electricity in medicine today involves variations on what goes by the name of transcutaneous neural stimulation — applying gel-coated electrodes to the surface of the skin to relieve pain, headaches, and even to treat drug addiction and withdrawal. Nobody can explain precisely how this works. Skin electrode units are a growth industry reimbursed by insurance policies around the world. Becker was one of the few voices to ask whether this growing application of electricity could have a dark side. He

175

questioned whether turning on the growth and healing in bones could safely be assumed not to turn on cells that might best be left alone.

Forgot Something?

Of course, there are many different types of electromagnetic exposure, reflecting the large array of uses of the vast spectrum of wavelengths and power densities.

If you think cell phones affect your health and I ask you to tell me about it, you can provide a sincere personal report. But from a scientific point of view the validity of your individual account cannot be assumed. One technique for evaluating whether there are immediate impacts of cell phone radiation on humans involves what is termed *blinding* — where both those being studied and those studying them do not know whether exposures to such radiation have taken place.

Dr. Stephan Braune of the University Neurology Clinic in Freiburg, Germany, carried out just such a blinded study in 1998 with ten volunteers. This work was published in the world's oldest medical journal, *The Lancet*. The Freiburg team used remote control devices that switched cell phones on or off when the volunteers held phones next to their heads. None of those being tested knew if the phones were emitting electromagnetic radiation or not. Much to the surprise of the investigators, each time the phones were turned on, blood pressure rose between five and ten millimeters. For most healthy people, this small change in blood pressure is of no consequence. But this level of increase could prove life-threatening in those who already have high blood pressure and could trigger a deadly heart attack or a stroke.

One study does not a revolution make. But it turns out that a blinded study was done — more than twenty years earlier. A senior navy researcher from Pensacola, Dietrich Beischer, had shown in 1973 that radio frequency signals raised triglycerides and blood pressure in humans. Just before he was to appear at a scientific meeting to discuss and expand upon these results, Becker reported that Beischer called him and blurted out in his German-accented voice:

"I'm at a pay phone. I can't talk long. They are watching me. I can't come to the meeting or ever communicate with you again. I'm sorry. You've been a good friend. Good-bye."

Beischer has never revealed who was watching him that day or what exactly had frightened him so much. But his work was all but forgotten. Virtually no one who read Braune's report would have remembered it, and the leader of the *Lancet* study in 1998 would not have been able to find it anywhere in the published literature. Beischer's work was carried out for the Office of Naval Research and according to the rules of the road at that time, others determined whether and whatever of his work would be published in the open literature. It never appeared outside the narrow confines of the Department of Defense, until I unearthed it four decades later.

Alzheimer's is one of the most dreaded diseases of the elderly. Named for the physician who first described the syndrome more than a century ago, it is in almost all cases not inherited, but a random event. Aside from repeated concussions from boxing or other rough sports, few causes of this disabling dementia have been identified. The first signs of Alzheimer's appear as nothing more than forgetfulness and memory lapses, the sorts of things that happen to anyone under stress who moves too quickly and forgets where she put her shopping list or glasses. In fact, the disease itself occurs when the brain loses critical neurons, and at its advanced state the imaging of the demented brain shows entire areas that are missing critical brain cells.

While we have about a hundred billion neurons, we cannot afford to lose half of them. Scans of the brains of those with Alzheimer's reveal that they have smaller working brains than normal people and that they develop unusual amounts of sticky gummed up residues within their brains — called beta amyloid plaques. Like our DNA, this particular plaque consists of nucleic acids, the basic building blocks of living matter. But unlike those of our DNA, the nucleic acids of plaque have gone amok. Rather than keeping a tightly wound order, amyloid plaques become tangled. Think of what happens to your undershirts or sheets if you don't take them out of the dryer right away and fold them neatly. They become jumbled and wrinkled. That's what amyloid plaques do to normal brain proteins as well, leaving a snarled mess of neurons and axons that lose their ability to connect properly. While all of us will develop some of these misfolded proteins if we live long enough, the brains of those with Alzheimer's are riddled with them.

A recent study of mice in the *Journal of Alzheimer's Disease*, 2010, received much attention. Some headlines were ecstatic. "Cell Phones Cure Alzheimer's!" Others questioned the results. "Could Cell Phones Cure Alzheimer's Disease?" Within three days the study summary had made it around the world, garnering front page coverage. Dr. Gary Arendash of the University of South Florida in Tampa was reported to have exposed both normal mice and a specially bred type of mouse that is prone to develop an Alzheimer's-like syndrome to cell phone radiation for two hours a day for nine months. In both types of animals, the cell-phone-exposed mice appeared to be smarter. In those bred to have dementia, exposure reversed the deposition of destructive amyloid protein that is the defining characteristic of the illness, and in normal mice such radiation appeared to sharpen memory.

The exposure set-up did not closely resemble a person holding a cell phone to his head. The exposure was in the far-field (instead of the near-field plume), and there was no magnetic field from the battery-current pulses. The researchers used a remote GSM simulator to produce the microwave signals. The media publicity from the university and others incorrectly stated "cell phones" — almost certainly industry-driven PR. The two electronic engineers who designed the exposure system are, surprisingly, not named as coauthors. One of them (Dr. Arsian) previously worked as an engineer at Ericsson.

Of course, we cannot conduct experiments on humans in the hope of learning whether cell phone radiation damages their brains, and we cannot look inside the brain after people talk on the phone to see how their brains have responded. Nonetheless, with so many of us using cell phones in so many ways, there are many "natural experiments" to evaluate, and it will take the next thirty years to complete that work.

At this point, psychiatrist Scott Mendelson finds the claims of a clear benefit against Alzheimer's for humans from cell phones based on this one study in rats vastly overstated. In the *Huffington Post*, in January 2010, Mendelson noted that, contrary to what the headlines implied, "unless you are using your cell phone to call your doctor for a good checkup or to buy a membership in a health club, that phone will not protect you from developing Alzheimer's disease."

The Sports Story You Haven't Heard

For more than three decades, Sam Milham worked as state epidemiologist in Seattle, Washington, turning official records of deaths and occupations into seminal and important work. Milham has produced impressive, original analyses showing that women and men who work in various jobs tend to die more often than others of some types of cancer and other chronic diseases. His work first showed that men who worked around high levels of electricity, such as power line men, or with electric power generation, had unusually high rates of brain cancer, non-Hodgkin's lymphoma, and breast cancer — the latter a disease that rarely affects men otherwise. In a recent paper in the journal *Medical Hypotheses*, Milham wondered whether there could be any common cause behind the fact that some professional athletes who had earned their living depending on their bodies to remain in peak condition had succumbed to one of the most dreaded nervous system diseases in the world. He reasoned that there could be a direct connection between the use of gently warming microwaves for diathermy treatment, transcutaneous neural stimulation and other electrical devices commonly used to treat pain in sports, and the onset of the disabling deadly degeneration of the nervous system known as Lou Gehrig's disease or amyotrophic lateral sclerosis (ALS).

This is a rare disease, but it appears to be becoming less rare today, especially among the young.

Lou Gehrig's disease usually strikes more men than women and affects those between the ages of forty and sixty. Based on past patterns, we know that half of all those affected by the disease die within three years. Only one in ten who develop this disabling degenerative disease has any family history of it. This means that, as with most cancers, nine out of ten cases of ALS occur in someone with no inherited risks, and are what is called sporadic. *Sporadic* is a term that signals we really have no idea whatsoever what may have caused the illness to occur. It could be just bad luck, a rotten roll of the dice of life, a random event, but we use the term sporadic to indicate that we are sure that it's definitely not bad genes inherited from one's parents.

Milham thinks he may know why more young and athletic people are developing Lou Gehrig's disease — a disease that resembles Parkinson's and Alzheimer's in its crippling impact on the nervous system and the body. He also thinks he may be able to explain why three out of fifty-five members of the 1964 San Francisco 49ers U.S. professional football team have died from exactly this disease so far, at much younger ages than most cases. Matt Hazeltine played more seasons with the 49ers at inside linebacker than anybody else in team history. Captain of the team for five seasons, he played in two Pro Bowls. He died from Lou Gehrig's disease at age fifty-three in 1987. Quarterback Bob Waters became coach and athletic director — a position that may well have put him in the training room where diathermy and other electronic devices were heavily used. Diagnosed with the disease at age forty-four, he died of Lou Gehrig's six years later. Fullback Gary Lewis died of the disease the same year he was diagnosed at age fifty-three. Other National Football League players who developed Lou Gehrig's disease include: O. J. Brigance, Glenn Montgomery, Steve Smith, Pete Duranko, Orlando Thomas, and Wally Hilgenberg.

Three is a small number, of course. The question is do these three persons have something in common that makes them a cohort, or is this merely a random occurrence — a cluster — that happened due to chance alone? What epidemiologists like Milham do is put this number in context by comparing the rate of this disease within the small group or cohort to which each man belonged with that found in the general population. To do this you need to know that the typical occurrence of ALS in the general population is 2.4 cases for every 100,000 people. Over a three-decade period of time, if you followed the health of 55 people of the ages of the 49er team members, you would expect less than one case to occur — in fact, the expected number is not a real one but .04 cases. Thus, the three cases in this team actually constitute seventy-five times the expected rate, a number that is generated by dividing the three actual cases by the expected rate of .04.

Another even more baffling instance of medical history reported by Milham was that of Melissa Jo Erickson, a twenty-six-year-old star basketball player for the University of Washington Huskies, diagnosed with ALS. At Heritage High School in Littleton, Colorado, the six-foot-three Ericson lettered all four years. After playing for the Huskies, she went on to play pro basketball in Europe. In 2007, her world crashed. She was diagnosed with Lou Gehrig's disease, at half the age of the typical case. Erickson told Milham that she had extensively used transcutaneous neural stimulation and other electrical devices to manage pain and various sports injuries throughout her decade-long basketball career.

Public health professionals seek to make order out of what looks like random events. The journal Neurology recently reported that slim, intense athletes develop Lou Gehrig's disease more often than their couch potato counterparts. Another report from the National Institutes of Health, published in *Annals of Neurology*, observed that persons with Lou Gehrig's disease tend to have abnormal lipids. Perhaps these two facts are linked? The common connection could well relate to exposure to diathermy and other electrical devices used to treat common athletic injuries. Several reports confirm that exposure to electromagnetic radiation elevates triglycerides, which in turn affect levels of fat in the blood. Could electromagnetic radiation damage the tight junctions that protect nerves throughout the body, just as it damages the blood-brain barrier in animals, and contribute to the onset of Lou Gehrig's disease? It turns out that the great Lou Gehrig himself was repeatedly treated by the team chiropractor to high levels of diathermy — the sort that could burn the leg, as it did to Joe DiMaggio and Babe Ruth.

While each case of any illness and each birth and each death is unique, the real work of public health is in discerning patterns that these create over time and in space. What we know is that Lou Gehrig's disease remains an enigma; it is increasingly afflicting the young along with professional athletes. The illness usually progresses rapidly and leads to death as the body loses the ability to control the muscles that allow movement, thinking, and breathing. As muscles stop being able to send or receive messages, they weaken, waste away, and twitch. Eventually the brain loses the ability to control the body. When muscles in the diaphragm and chest wall fail, individuals require mechanical support just to breathe. Usually, Lou Gehrig's disease does not impair the mind. But some victims may lose their ability to think clearly, to remember important things, may eventually suffer full dementia — much as happens with Alzheimer's.

Remembering The Electric Doctor

Today a vibrant research community is working on the use of electromagnetic currents to heal bone, relieve aches and pains, carry out surgical procedures, and even regenerate damaged spinal cords and brains. Sadly, Becker, whose findings laid the framework for much of the work using bioelectromagnetic stimulation on limb and spinal cord regeneration, and those who worked closely with him, like researcher Andrew Marino, were unable to complete their studies.

Having documented the ways that small amounts of current affected bone metabolism and limb regrowth, Becker became convinced that the way electricity was generated and transported through high-voltage switching stations could put people at risk. When New York State was considering major expansions of high voltage power lines, including placing them directly above public schools and playgrounds, Becker spoke out, arguing that some forms of electric power generation and transmission could endanger public health.

Louis Slesin, the iconoclastic editor of *Microwave News*, who has tracked every major story on this topic for nearly a quarter of a century, praises Becker as "the most important electromagnetic spectrum scientist of this era. . . . He was a real scientist, unlike many of the people in the field. He did research and was light-years ahead of everybody else. The whole problem with the benefits of tissue healing and regeneration, as with all medical applications, is the other side of the coin — negative health effects. People don't want to accept the idea that electricity has such strong impacts on biology.

"When David Carpenter [a doctor directing the New York State Public Health investigation of the matter] took on the issue of power lines for New York State in the 1980s, he basically did not believe there was any problem at all and he said so. What makes Carpenter so unique is that, like Becker, he remains a very serious scientist who was moved by the data. When Carpenter took a good hard look at the information that Becker and others had amassed on the potential of power lines to impact the body, he actually changed his own view. To the surprise of many, New York State restrained some of the expansions of power lines.

"From his years of meticulous work Becker understood, in ways that few others did, that electricity had powerful and direct effects on the body. People simply did not want to think about the logical implications of all this, especially given how hugely profitable various parts of the industry remain."

At this point, Slesin is jaded. "You run into non sequiturs all over the place. It's all a very weird disconnect. On the one hand, you have the FDA approving all sorts of applications like bone healing stimulators because they can clearly be beneficial, although nobody can tell us precisely how they work. On the other hand, when scientists like Becker raise the specter of what this could mean for our long-term health and the growth of cells we do not need, the same agency that approves the use of electricity for medical purposes claims that it is just impossible for these electromagnetic signals or for cell phone radiation to have any negative impact on human health."

Slesin is a true muckraker in the tradition of I. F. Stone, the progressive journalist, and Upton Sinclair, whose searing exposé of the meatpacking industry in *The Jungle* spurred the federal government to set standards for foods and drugs. The editor and publisher of the only independent trade voice on microwaves in the world, Microwave News, Slesin still is not sure whether cell phones are dangerous. But he certainly knows that their safety has not been proved. Slesin has been working on this issue so long, and seen so many promising leads shot down by scientists for hire, that he's become cynical.

"The thing that keeps you going in this business is that serious scientists like Becker, Carpenter, Abe Liboff, Jerry Phillips, and Lennart Hardell keep pushing the work ahead. I used to think things would change when we had clear evidence. But now I realize that this may never happen. Even if you do get the dead bodies, it won't be enough. It won't happen. There's just too much money involved. Is that optimistic enough for you?"

In fact, in the bone healing business, Slesin recalls that a number of the scientists were at each others' throats. The company Electro-Biology, Inc., which was formed eventually by Drs. Andrew Bassett and Arthur Pilla, made a lot of money. Robert Becker was the one who admitted that nobody could yet explain precisely how electrical stimulation worked to promote bone healing, and he remained deeply interested in the basic science. He and these others had different points of view regarding commercial opportunities. As he relates in his own account of his life work, *The Body Electric*, Becker found himself cut off from funding to study the basic biology of bone healing, and how electromagnetic radiation impacted the body, at precisely the time when he became outspoken about the potential hazards of power lines. The two types of exposure are radically different, the one involving low frequency electromagnetic fields, the other using various frequencies of even lower exposures. But it made no sense to Becker to assume that the only biological impacts of any exposure were either positive or nothing at all.

Becker may have become a hero to parents of children whose schools would have fallen directly under proposed routes of power lines in New York State, but in the end he paid a heavy price. His laboratories, which had been in business for thirty years, lost all their funding. People who had collaborated with him for years suddenly stopped talking to him. Here's how he ended his memoir, recalling this 1985 calamity:

I want the general public to know that science isn't run the way they read about it in the newspapers and magazines. I want laypeople to understand that they cannot automatically accept scientists' pronouncements at face value, for too often they're self-serving and misleading. I want our citizens, nonscientists as well as investigators, to work to change the way research is administered. The way it's currently funded and evaluated, we're learning more and more and about less and less, and science is becoming our enemy instead of our friend.

9

PUBLIC HEALTH ISN'T PHYSICS

Can't fall asleep? Can't stay awake? Dizzy? Feeling fogged or stoned without pot or drugs? Blurred vision and dulled hearing? Jumping thoughts? Buzzing brain? Moving fast and forgetting where you are going? Stuttering and losing your train of thought? Misplaced your ATM card? Can't find the remote control again? Forgot to pick up your dry cleaning and where you parked your car? Don't know why you keep yelling at your wife? Lost your bike lock key inside the laundry bag? Perhaps you are simply a bit stressed.

We all know that the modern world is jam-packed with so much happening all at once that many of us lose it from time to time. When a person is afflicted with what could simply be the result of too much work and too little sleep, the last thing one wonders is whether our brains have stopped working well because something is growing inside our heads that does not belong. Brain tumors sleep within our bodies, growing slowly until they announce themselves in an irrefutable manner — often through a major epileptic seizure or a sudden clot of blood in the brain that produces a stroke. A brain tumor is a hypochondriac's worst fear and everyone's absolute nightmare. Even those who know little about their bodies understand that cancer and the brain simply do not mix. Our thick skulls are not made to expand. Tumors of the head are usually fatal and horrible.

How Can You Predict a Tumor?

Solving the puzzle of why any particular person gets brain cancer is not something that can easily be done today. The study of what causes brain tumors is one of the toughest jobs in epidemiology. As one of the core fields of study in public health, epidemiology studies the past in an attempt to make the future healthier. Epidemiologists look at patterns of disease as they occur in many people over time in an effort to identify things that can be done to change those patterns in the future. Brain cancer can take several decades to develop. We know this today, because of studies that have been carried out over the past half century. The Hiroshima and Nagasaki bombings that ended World War II killed around two hundred thousand people within a few months. But studies of the thousands who survived the atomic bombing in 1945 have left little doubt about another tragic consequence. Forty years after the single blast of ionizing radiation from the bomb, people who survived have double the risk of brain tumors compared to those who did not experience that exposure.

Remember the people I mentioned in chapter 5 who had suffered seizures? That epidemiological discovery about ionizing radiation and atomic bomb survivors does not apply to them. Alan Marks's world crashed at two in the morning the night before he and his wife, Ellie, were set to go to their youngest child's college graduation.

"At first I thought he was having a very bad dream. I tried to shake him. I shouted, 'Alan!! Alan?? Alan??' I couldn't wake him up," said Ellie.

Alan was taken by ambulance to a local hospital, where a scan of his head revealed what had triggered this convulsive seizure of the brain. Inside the right side of his forehead sat a golfball-size tumor. He had a cancerous mass (oligodendroglioma). Doctors told the Marks family the grim news. His children were dumbstruck but also in a strange way relieved. Suddenly years of baffling behavior made sense. He had not in fact stopped loving them, even though he had treated them insufferably. The tumor had invaded the part of his brain that controls affection and tenderness.

"We had entered a living nightmare. Alan had always been pretty healthy. But for several years his behavior had become stranger and stranger. When you love someone your entire life and he begins to become another person, to act strangely against those they hold dear, you try with all your heart to find ways to help."

Fast, smart, and driven, with an ironic sense of humor and timing, Alan had become cruel and forgetful, lashing out at those around him without provocation. Psychiatrists had declared Alan bipolar and prescribed various medications, and intense family therapy. For a while that diagnosis seemed to make sense. After all, Alan certainly had huge mood swings and could sometimes get by on little sleep. He could still be utterly charming or astonishingly vicious. The family resigned themselves to working through the diagnosis, despite the outbursts and unpredictable actions.

When the tumor was finally diagnosed, Ellie began to grasp what lay behind some of Alan's awful behavior. "The right frontal lobe where his tumor originated is the core of empathy, knowing the difference between right and wrong, and many other personality and cognitive functions."

As the family struggled with the bleak prospects, they learned that

Alan was not alone. Just ten days after Alan got the devastating news, Senator Ted Kennedy had a major convulsive seizure and faced the very same diagnosis — a glioma of the brain.

The Markses' son Zack had just finished interning with the senator. He remembered the hours he had seen the senator with his cell phone held next to his head. Zack had a sinking feeling that there might be some connection between his dad's diagnosis and that of Senator Kennedy. He soon learned that the Kennedy family had strong suspicions that the senator's tumor was in some way connected to his cell phone use. When Ellie heard this, suddenly it all made sense.

"For years, we used to joke about Alan and his cell phones. He had one of the first car phones, and then one of the first bag phones. As he worked deals around the area, he could not be separated from his phone. At one point, we drove back home several hours from a planned family vacation to pick up his phone that he had left behind. He was never, never away from one of those phones. He probably used various phones for at least ten thousand hours. My husband was and is one of the top real estate brokers in our region. The phone was his lifeline for his work."

Like Ellie, Mindy Brown and her husband, Dan, the defensive line coach for California State University at Fresno, the couple I also mentioned in chapter 5, had been high school sweethearts. Their house was command central for their own children, many friends, football players, and wannabes. Their six children included two who played for the Bulldogs, the Fresno team. Dan would be on the phone sometimes for four hours at a stretch when he traveled to Southern California to check out new recruits. Coach Brown's seizure occurred when he was talking on his phone in May 2007.

Mindy recalls, "There was one phone in particular that he complained would make his head and ear hurt when he spoke on it for more than several minutes. His right ear would be bright red where he had held his phone and his eye might hurt. He complained so much about his cell phone that I took it to Sprint to trade it for a different model, but because it was assigned to the university I was unable to do so. . . . Within a few months my husband went from knocking two-hundred-fifty-pound linebackers on their fannies during practice drills to patting them on their heads to console them as they knelt by his deathbed."

Who Killed My Husband?

The first thing a person asks after being told he or she has cancer is, "Why me?" All the publicity about brain tumors and cell phones has led many to grasp, and tightly hold, this explanation of the loss or misfortune of their loved one. *Ah, the cell phone did it. I'll hate cell phones for the rest of my life.* Simple. Even comforting.

Cancer patients' lives are taken over by medical appointments. They spend a lot of time waiting. Some folks cannot bear to talk. Mindy Brown got tired of hearing that her husband's doctors just were not sure why her once strong, healthy husband had developed such a deadly tumor. She began doing what she thought of as research.

Mindy is one of those people with a straightforward smile and direct manner whom you could imagine going into the lion's den and managing to make such amiable small talk the beasts would be charmed. Mindy and her son had traveled to Augusta, Maine, in the late winter of 2010, because they wanted the legislature to hear and see what brain cancer looked and felt like to those who had lost the center of their family. As Mindy sat in clinics waiting for reports and doctors' visits, she would notice lots of things. In the days and weeks after surgery, those who have had their heads shaved and drilled to remove tumors wear stretch caps to cover it all up. Opening with her warm smile, Mindy would quietly begin the conversation, "Hello. We're waiting to find out about Dan's tumor.

It was right next to his ear where he used his cell phone. Did you use a cell phone very often?"

"Every single person I asked had the same answer." Mindy remembered all this when we talked at the hearings in Augusta to consider putting labels on cell phones. "Yes. . . ."

After a while Dan got tired of this routine. "Look, honey, just stop. You know what the answer will be. Of course it's the phones."

But is there really any proof that cell phones cause brain tumors? This could all just be a coincidence created when saddened people desperately look for answers to questions that few are asking.

Mindy and Ellie do not pretend to be scientists. They are angry. When representatives of the cell phone industry point to the absence of an epidemic of brain tumors as proof of safety, they become livid. They have learned a lot about brain tumors and know that tumors only occur after decades when exposures to agents like cigarette smoke, asbestos, vinyl chloride, or benzene have been very, very high. The fact that any increase in tumor risk has shown up in heavy cell phone users after only one decade should be setting off alarm bells. Because their husbands were such heavy users and first adopters of the technology, they used older phones that operated at different levels of radio frequency radiation with different types of signals. They also appreciate how unusual their husbands were ten or fifteen years ago, when they began their heavy cell phone habits. And they know that just ten years ago fewer than one in three Americans used a cell phone and even fewer used phones as heavily as their husbands did then or as growing numbers of us do today. "Are we supposed to wait for more and more people to die like my Danny?" Mindy asks. "I just can't do that."

Dan made her promise to tell people why he and she and so many others became convinced that his brain tumor was not just bad luck, but the result of his thousands of hours of cell phone use. Mindy understands that because so few people have used cell phones for as long as her husband did, there could not possibly be a general epidemic of brain tumors now. "Is that really what we have to have happen? Have we learned nothing from tobacco?" she asked me when we talked about this during a break in the hearings in Maine, where she tried to tell people what had happened to Dan.

Mindy's subjective survey is not science. She knows that. Cell phones cannot be studied like drugs in a controlled trial. Given that brain cancer can take decades to develop, and that cell phone technology today is quite different from what it was a decade ago, how do we know if today's phones are better or worse? The Food and Drug Administration does not test cell phones for safety before they are marketed and does not monitor them for safety afterward but relies on the advice of the industry and proddings from consumer groups.

In The Long Run

Brain cancer can take forty years to develop and, like all cancers, can have many different causes. Some studies have found that eating smoked meats and hot dogs, or working with certain chlorinated cleaning compounds, may increase the risk of brain tumors some forty years later. Analyses of patterns of the disease in men and women who have repaired antennas or radar for three decades have established that they tend to have higher rates of brain cancer, some forms of leukemia, as well as unusually high rates of breast cancer in men.

When Alan Marks contacted Dr. Lennart Hardell, an expert in the field in Sweden, where cell and cordless phones have been used for much longer, Hardell told him that he thought it was more likely than not that Alan's tumor was associated with his ten thousand hours of cell phone use. More likely than not, that's how scientists talk. That's because we seldom can speak about direct causes of such a complicated disease as brain cancer.

193

When I spoke with Dr. Hardell, I asked him to explain how he could have reached this conclusion, since so many epidemiologists remained unsure that there is any connection between cell phones and brain tumors.

"We have to examine all the information we have. To me that means I do not merely consider whether we have enough human studies. After all, we know that those will take several more decades to complete. I look carefully at what we know from experiments with animals, short-term exposures to humans about their memory and other brain functions. Then we must combine this with observations we make by studying people with the disease and comparing them to those without it. In my studies I find one pattern over and over again. Those who have used their phones the most and for the longest, have more malignant brain tumors than others."

Unlike researchers in the United States and Canada, where regular use of phones is much more recent, Hardell has been able to study people who used phones extensively for a decade or more in Sweden. He has found that the heaviest users have doubled the risk of brain tumors after a decade. Hardell is not alone in coming up with this result. Similar findings have been developed by scientists in Israel, Finland, Russia, and England. Recently Hardell has also shown that those who start using cell phones regularly as teenagers have four times more brain cancer about ten years later.

Studying The Car In Which We Are Driving

Still, the cell phone industry repeats in 2010 what it said in 1993, when the first claims were made that cell phones could cause brain tumors. When, in September of 2009, Senators Tom Harkin of Iowa and Arlen Specter of Pennsylvania held the first hearing on the subject in three decades, the CTIA President and CEO Steve Largent issued the following statement:

"CTIA and the wireless industry are deeply committed to safety and to providing timely, accurate information to consumers about wireless phones. When it comes to the facts about cell phones and health-related effects, the industry relies on the conclusions of impartial groups such as the U.S. Food and Drug Administration (FDA), the World Health Organization (WHO), the American Cancer Society, and the National Institutes of Health, which have all concluded that the scientific evidence to date does not demonstrate any adverse health effects associated with the use of wireless phones."

How committed to "timely, accurate information" can the wireless association be if there is not now nor has there ever been a major research program in the U.S. government on cell phones? Motorola shut down its own laboratories two years ago. Of course, there is a program of classified military research, given the uses of wireless technology in warfare and weaponry and the need to protect our armed forces with fabrics, barriers, and devices, but there is no public program about the biological consequences of cell phones for the civilian population.

Industry responded to the first lawsuits on cell phones and brain cancer in 1993 by invoking ten thousand studies and forty years of research showing safety. At the time that assertion was made, it was at worst a lie and at best a profound distortion of reality. When that bogus claim was made, fewer than one in one hundred Americans owned a cell phone — some thirteen million people. The next year the number of cell phone subscribers had doubled. Concerned that bad news could harm the expanding market, industry declared its support in 1993 for what was billed as more research but was in fact the start of something new. In response to questions about safety, the CTIA began what became the twenty-eight-million-dollar Wireless Technology Research (WTR) program, led by George Carlo, an articulate lawyer-scientist. Carlo had formerly conducted defensive research for Dow Chemical, the Chlorine Chemistry Council, and Philip Morris, and had no experience at all with radio frequency radiation.

While Carlo may have started out as one of industry's own, he ended up in quite another camp seven years later when he sounded alarms about the invisible hazards of the wireless age — the subtitle of the book he wrote with the investigative journalist Martin Schram in 2001. When the WTR began to show that cell phone radiation could be dangerous, Carlo reports that he was basically fired. Photos from his book show Carlo fishing, golfing, and engaging in other high-end activities on expeditions with Tom Wheeler, then chief of the CTIA, and other industry luminaries. Louis Slesin, the acerbic editor of *Microwave News*, doesn't buy the story line that Carlo suddenly turned his back on the finer things in life when he discovered the dangers of cell phone radiation. Not mincing words, Slesin calls Carlo "a con man hired to give the appearance that something was being done when it was not." In 2003, *Microwave News* claimed that

> *Carlo and the industry he represented never wanted to do any actual research. . . . WTR's $25-million research budget was by far the largest pot of money ever earmarked for RF research. It was squandered. . . . By dangling a huge amount of money in front of the cash-starved radio-frequency research community, Carlo guaranteed silent obedience. Anyone who dared complain risked being cut off from his millions. There was the added benefit that scientists were discouraged from helping lawyers who were thinking about suing cell phone companies.*

Slesin is clearly no fan of Carlo. "What Carlo did was unspeakable. After 2001, he wrote these letters to the CEOs of every telecom company changing sides, warning them about the dangers of their products. I have a document where he pitches to do WTR 2, asking for the grand sum of fifty million dollars. . . . Having failed to hold them up for any more money to continue extending the fruitless WTR, he got vindictive and went public with his criticisms of the industry."

Slesin charges that after expending all those industry funds and having so little to show for it, Carlo is like the man who shoots his parents and then complains he is an orphan. Carlo vehemently denies these charges using language that is not suitable for this book. Whatever may have been the motivation for Carlo's conversion from cell phone industry advocate to cell phone activist, there is no denying that there is little scientific literature to show for the millions that were spent on the WTR, aside from a summary of some of that work that appears in Carlo's book. There is also no denying that in his public statements and publications since then, Carlo has sounded everlouder alarms. There may be nothing more furious than a scientist scorned. Since Carlo parted ways with the CTIA, he has produced an astonishingly brutal series of statements indicting the industry.

Carlo claims that the distinguished and prolific former National Cancer Institute scientist John D. Boice offered expert services to the WTR as a way to neutralize the brain tumor connection. It is next to impossible to know what really happened. The International Epidemiology Institute (IEI) did work with the Danish Cancer Society on cell phones and brain tumors. But Carlo also claims that the IEI profited from this effort. Boice denies this. He told Paul Goldberg, editor of *The Cancer Letter*, that no money was ever received by the IEI for doing research with the Danish Cancer Society on cell phones. The IEI contribution, which was substantial, was made solely as an investment in future work. Indeed, the Danish Cancer Society did in fact collaborate with the IEI in producing a widely publicized study that found no increased risk of brain tumors tied with cell phone use.

That study appeared to great acclaim. Headlines around the world boasted of this latest finding from an impeccable source published in a first-tier scientific journal, the *Journal of the National Cancer Institute*, where Boice had for years had a distinguished record.

These good news headlines appeared within days of publication:

- "CELL PHONES DON' T CAUSE BRAIN CANCER"
  — *Toronto Daily News, December 10, 2006*
- "CELL PHONES DON' T RAISE CANCER RISK"
  — *Reuters, December 6, 2006*
- "BIG STUDY FINDS NO LINK BETWEEN CELL PHONES, CANCER"
  — *San Jose Mercury News, December 6, 2006*
- "STUDY: CELL PHONES SAFE"
- — *Newsday*, December 7, 2006
- "CELL PHONES DO NOT CAUSE CANCER"
  — *Techtree.com, India, December 7, 2006*

After this result was so widely publicized, Carlo reported that "Boice went on a bit of a television tour to blunt the effects of my just published exposé on the topic — 'Cell Phones: Invisible Hazards in the Wireless Age.' The reason for Boice's television tour was simple. My book created big waves and big concerns. Dr. Boice provided an antidote to the issues I was raising. I faced off with him a couple of times on TV."

In this highly touted Danish study, let's look at what the researchers actually did.

They reviewed health records through 2002 of about 421,000 people who had first signed up for private use of cell phones between 1982 and 1995. A "cell phone user" in the study was anyone who made a single phone call a week for six months during the period

1981 to 1995. The study kicked out about 200,000 people — anyone who was part of a business that used cell phones — and included only those who had used a cell phone for personal purposes for eight years. Think of those early clunker phones with their battery packs, cumbersome cords, and hefty monthly fees and how rarely people used phones back in the early days.

This research design raises a lot of questions. Why did they not look at business users — those with far more frequent use of cell phones? Why lump all users together, putting those who might have made a single cell phone call a week with those who used the phones more often? Why stop collecting information on brain tumors in 2002? Use of cell phones has grown more than fourfold since then in many countries.

When you are looking at a large population to find an effect, generally the more people you study, the better your chance of finding something. But if you include lots of people without much exposure alongside those with very high exposure, you dilute the high-exposure group and so lower your chances of finding any effect at all. Lumping all these various users together is like looking all over a city for a stolen car, when you know it's within a five-block radius. Perhaps you'll find what you're looking for, but the chances are greater that you won't. The Danish study was designed to look definitively thorough — 421,000 people! — but in fact it was biased against positive findings from the start.

If you want to find out whether cell phone use causes brain cancer, the higher the use or exposure of those you are examining, the better the odds that you will be able to find whether it's made a difference. It's clear that the early analog phones must be different from the newer digital ones. We hope the difference is big and that those of us using phones today face a lowered risk, but we have no way to know whether this is the case. Some believe that using earpieces connected by wires should reduce our direct exposures, but, again, evidence on this is not at hand. Bluetooth systems substantially reduce the amount of radio frequency radiation into the brain compared to holding the phone up to your head.

But if the phone to which Bluetooth is connected is kept directly on the body, then exposures will still be and risks may also mount. People keep Bluetooth in their ears all day long and the power levels have increased since Bluetooth first came out.

In all circumstances, research works best when we have solid information on the nature of use or exposure we are looking at. All of us have cell phone bills that provide detailed records of our use, and most of these can be accessed online. These were not used in this study, or in any study of the industry to date. A gold mine of data lies untapped.

The Danish study, as the headlines made clear, found no increase in risk of brain cancer for private users of cell phones. The reason the researchers were looking for brain cancer is straightforward. As the authors noted, cell phone signals do penetrate the brain. "During operation, the antenna of a cellular telephone emits radio frequency electromagnetic fields that can penetrate 4–6 cm into the human brain."

Despite the work of Frey, Lai, Gandhi, and others, along with Adlkofer's recent, quite substantial confirmation of biological damage, a vibrant debate continues over what the radiation absorption of microwaves means biologically. How much of this debate is genuine and how much is mostly manufactured by those seeking to prolong doubt cannot easily be determined at this point. Peer review and doing science when more than a trillion-dollar global industry is involved becomes a daunting, often perilous enterprise.

We know that cell phone signals enter the side of the head, where the auditory nerve sits, and also enter the cheek where the parotid gland is located. An earlier Swedish analysis compared more than fourteen hundred people with brain tumors to a similar number without the disease from 1997 to 2000 — more than ten years ago. They found that tumors of the auditory nerve were three times more frequent in persons who had used cell phones for more than a decade. In 2004, other Swedish researchers reported that long-term users had significantly more tumors on the auditory nerves than nonusers. One study that was well publicized in 2000 found no increased risk of brain cancer in cell phone users; but the average person in this widely publicized study had used a phone for less than three years. Still, even within this limited study there was an intriguing fact. Those who had used phones for this short period of time had twice the risk of a very rare brain tumor — neuroepitheliomatous cancers — the kind that wraps itself around the nerve cells of the lining of the brain, right at the locus that cell signals can reach.

The problems these studies are trying to understand are inherently complex. Science works best studying one thing at a time, as we do with drugs in clinical trials. The problems posed by cell phones in the real world are like huge simultaneous equations — mathematical formulas of relationships between multiple unknowns. How can you determine the role of one factor, such as cell phone exposure to the skull, when all others, like diet, workplace conditions, and local air pollution, are changing at the same time and at different rates? Given how broadly cell phone signals now penetrate our worlds of the coffee shop, airports, and some downtown areas of major cities, where do we find any truly unexposed groups to compare results against? Moreover, the study of chronic health problems is complicated by the assumption that a single condition gave rise to a single outcome, even though we know that life is seldom so simple. Because cell phone use has grown so fast and technologies change every year, it is as if we are trying to study the car in which we are driving.

The studies Carlo and other scientists never published for the industry began as a series of projects looking into whether cell phone signals disrupted cultures of living animal cells grown in the laboratory. Human studies zeroed in on brain cancer — a relatively rare but often fatal disease. Some of the work done in laboratories clearly showed that wireless signals could affect the ways cells talk to one another to stay under control — what is called gap-junction communication. Under healthy conditions, cells send messages through proteins and enzymes that keep things in order and tell badly behaving cells to get in line or die. Wireless signals were shown to disturb this ability. Cells that can't communicate well are prone to grow out of control. In essence, the wireless signals promoted a kind of social breakdown among cells.

Other experimental studies produced solid biological grounds for thinking that pulsed microwave radiation has important impacts of precisely the sort that can lead to cancer. This included a series of studies showing precancerous microscopic changes in exposed cells and a weakened blood-brain barrier in living animals. The way all this could lead to cancer is straightforward. First, a breakdown in the barrier that normally protects the brain allows whatever pollutants are already in the body (as a result of being alive in the modern world) to enter into sensitive tissue that is not well-protected. Once these foreign agents get into the brain or on to the nerves, they then can wreak the sort of havoc on DNA that is evidenced in animal studies, including damage to the ability of cells to repair themselves. Unrepaired cells cannot defend themselves against the ordinary assaults of life and are therefore primed to become cancerous.

At the core of the WHO Interphone study of three thousand brain tumors in thirteen different countries is a major effort to learn from patients whether they used cell phones more frequently than did others. The limits of the work are easy to grasp. The ways to overcome them are not. The results were just published as this book was going to press.

Today it would be hard to find many adults who do not use a cell phone. But when the Interphone study was being carried out from 2000 to 2004, people who did not use cell phones very much at all were compared with those who developed two types of brain tumors: gliomas and meningiomas. Gliomas are highly malignant tumors that begin in the glial cells of the brain, the nonpulsing cells that support the neurons and hold them together. Their growth can be silent, with symptoms that mimic flu or a headache. But eventually, they become undeniable. Both Alan Marks and Dan Brown developed types of gliomas. Marks recovered. Brown did not. Meningiomas are technically considered benign tumors, because they do not necessarily kill you. They arise within the meninges that protect the spinal cord and brain. But meningiomas can recur and can also become fatal, depending on where they occur and how big they are before they are removed. People can lose speech, sight, movement, or hearing, depending on where the tumor starts and where it ends up. Lloyd Morgan recovered from his meningioma fifteen years ago.

The Interphone published analyses so far describe the personal experiences of 5,117 gliomas and meningiomas that occurred in people ages thirty to fifty-nine who lived in thirteen industrial nations between 2000 and 2004 and were compared to a similar number of controls who had used cell phones five hours a month or less. When interviewed on the day after brain surgery to remove their tumors, less than one in ten reported heavy cell phone use in 1990 through 1994. About 10 percent of those with brain tumors in the Interphone study reported talking on their phone without a hands-free device for a total of more than 1,640 hours. An even smaller proportion indicated that they made more than 27,000 calls in their lifetime.

In looking at the persons who agreed to serve as controls, it becomes apparent that most of them had some use of a cell phone.

This is why the lowest level of use in both the cases and controls is referred to as "never regular user," rather than as "no user." Even at the time the Interphone study was carried out some ten years ago, there were few people who never used a cell phone. Interestingly, more than half of those asked to participate as controls at the same time between 2000 and 2004 refused to do so. A user of a cell phone was defined as an individual who made just one call a week for six months. If a person used a hands-free device, she was assumed to have had no exposures to radio frequency at all for the amount of time such a device was used. The use of cordless home telephones, which also emit radio frequency radiation quite similar to that of cell phones, was also not considered.

It certainly looks like the cases in this study were unusual in many ways. One stands out especially — the average use of a cell phone by men and women diagnosed with malignant glioma in the Interphone study was about one hundred hours, about ninety minutes a month, or about two thousand calls in an entire lifetime. Thus, this means that the Interphone study ended up comparing people who used cell phones just a little bit, with those who used cell phones a bit more — say, twenty times more. But these numbers pale by comparison to today, when ordinary use has skyrocketed.

Alan Marks and Dan Brown used cell phones ten times as much, if not more, than the average person with brain cancer in the Interphone study. Many teenagers and young adults talk on their phones today at similar levels, although growing numbers are texting. Today in America, the average cell phone bill in many urban areas is for one to three thousand minutes a month — about 160 hours to 480 hours. Some teenagers and young adults reportedly are on their phones for more than six hours a day. The Interphone study included no young adults, no teenagers, and no children — the groups in whom usage is increasing most around the world. In America half of all eight-year-olds have a cell phone, as do three out of every four twelve-year-olds.

The conclusions of the Interphone study are fascinating and limited, as the authors acknowledge. In fact, regular cell phone users in this study, who used phones modestly compared to today, actually have fewer brain tumors than the controls with whom they are compared. The authors acknowledge that they cannot explain this unless perhaps radio frequency radiation actually does protect against brain tumors, maybe for a while. If one looks at the relatively small number of people in the Interphone study that were the greatest cell phone talkers, those who reported using phones heavily for ten years have about a doubled risk of developing a glioma on the same side of the head they recall having used their phone. For meningioma, the highest users actually had more than four times the risk of the not-regular users when their uses of both the old-fashioned analog and digital phones were combined.

Whatever these results may portend for public health, the growth of cell phones is poised to enter yet another revolutionary phase, according to Mary Meeker, dubbed by *Barron's* the queen of the Net.

The Morgan Stanley analyst told the annual Google gaggle in March 2010 that the world is currently in the midst of the fifth major technology cycle of the past half century. The first cycle began with building-size mainframe computers of the 1950s and 1960s that had to be fed keypunched cards that were counter-sorted into results printed out on huge rolls of punched paper. The introduction of the smaller desktop computers of the 1970s and Internet connections to computers of the 1980s formed the second and third cycles, with more streamlined outputs on screens and printers. We are ending the fourth era now with the expansion of the mobile Internet and digitized output directly into computers, GPS, televisions, and the like. Meeker believes that within the next five years "more users will connect to the Internet over mobile devices than desktop PCs." As she puts it on one of the slides in the report released to Google's annual Las Vegas celebration: "Rapid Ramp of Mobile Internet Usage Will Be a Boon to Consumers and Some Companies Will Likely Win Big (Potentially Very Big) While Many Will Wonder What Just Happened."

One in five people around the world today has access to the faster 3G network, which relies on more powerful pulsed signals. None of these changes could be incorporated into the Interphone study, of course. Nor does Interphone shed any light on what, if anything, this phenomenal increase in use may mean for our health.

Although the Interphone study stopped gathering cases and was completed when former director Brundtland had promised in 2005, it did not appear until five years after it was finished. No reasons have been offered for this delay. That study was not designed to deal with the spread of this technology. With nearly all adults using cell phones today, we have lost any pretense of a control group.

The delay in releasing the Interphone results is unsurprising, given the disconnect that exists between our enthralled use of the technology, and the nagging sense by many experts that there is a need to be smarter about how we use it. Some German findings published in 2009 are especially disquieting. The German study captured information about the daily lives of people in Mainz, Bielefeld, and Heidelberg. What did they have for breakfast regularly? Where did they live? How often did they use the cell phone? For how long? On which ear? These are the sorts of things epidemiologists like me hope you remember. This work contrasted the life experiences and reported cell phone use of 366 people with deadly tumors of the brain called gliomas and 381 with slow-growing, usually benign tumors of the membranes that cover the spinal cord, against some 1,500 people between the ages of thirty and sixty-nine who had better luck and did not have brain tumors. When asking both groups about their past and current uses of cell phones, they did not find any increased risk in those who used phones for less than a decade. That was not the end of this work, however, but merely the start.

In this same study, those who reported having used cell phones for ten years or more had twice the risk of gliomas — just like Interphone has found, just like Hardell and other researchers have shown. It should be obvious that looking at people with a fatal illness and asking them to try hard to remember, in some cases, what they did up to forty years ago is not easy. With all the information governments now assemble to combat terror, including library and cell phone records, how hard could it be to learn whether our use of cell phones places us at risk from a disease that could be averted through better design and technology?

Epidemiological studies to date that have not found a general, clear, and consistent risk from cell phones have, for the most part, looked at older technologies over short periods of exposure. And none has asked about the impact of cell phones on the brains of children and teenagers. Excepting Hardell, few have examined the impact of cordless phones. Don't we want to know? Don't we need to know? Don't we have a right to know?

To say there is a powerful force clearing the way for the continued awesome growth of the cell phone industry is putting it mildly. Perhaps no tale makes this as glaringly clear as one from George Carlo about Joshua Muscat. Remember, no facts here are in dispute.

Muscat worked for Carlo in the WTR, carrying out a case control study of brain tumors and cell phone use. In the first report that Muscat gave on this work there was a small but significant increase in specific tumors of the neuroepithelium on the same side of the head that cell phone use had been reported. Carlo writes:

The industry hired an epidemiologist named Linda Erdreich to participate in the peer review. Under her influence, Muscat's data "mysteriously" changed — not once, but twice. First, in

*the report Muscat gave at the Second State of the Science Collo-
quium — and published in the book that contains all of the papers
presented at the Long Beach Colloquium in June 1999 — the
statistically significant correlation between the side of the head
where tumors were and the side of the head where phones were
used disappeared. Then, yet again, in the paper that he submitted to the Journal of the American Medical Association, the data
were further altered so that the statistically significant increase
in tumor risk disappeared as well. Both of these alterations in
the data were flagrant breaches of the peer-reviewed scientific
protocols that were intended to guide that research. In a letter
to the editor of JAMA before the study was published, I pointed
these inconsistencies out and indicated that I was the funder of
the study. The journal ignored the letter and went forward with
the publication. Clearly, the industry carefully orchestrated the
Muscat fraud so that the data that were "published" in JAMA
carried no statistical significance. The press release for that
study carried the "no statistical findings" heading. Of course,
all of these data manipulations are evident in published papers,
but no one has chosen to raise the issue in the media.*

Don't Ask, Can't Tell

Allan Frey, the researcher who, as a young man starting in the early
1960s, did original work sponsored by the Office of Naval Research,
showed that microwave radiation like that used in cell phones today
could weaken the membranes surrounding our hearts, brains, eyes,
and lungs. A Chinese proverb explains the response to this work: If
you do not want to know, don't ask. He said to me recently:

After my work appeared and others supported some of it,
effectively everything in the U.S. on these topics was shut down.

Today, you can't get funding to do anything of consequence. Even the military part of the program is closed, although I don't know about classified work. The one study that is being planned by the National Toxicology Program assumes that the effects of radio frequency radiation follows a dose-response curve like most toxic substances. In fact, it is not merely the intensity of the energy that is important. More important are the frequencies and modulations of the signals. It is the pulsed signals of digital phones today that are the issue and much more problematic biologically. We're going to spend millions of dollars and find nothing, if we fail to look at this and rely on a toxicant-based model that assumes a simple relationship where the greater the dose, the greater the response.

Frey may be retired from active research, but he remains an instructive critic. He bemoans the focus on brain cancer altogether, noting that it will take way too long to find out if there is a problem, at which point it will be too late for billions around the world.

"We need to stop looking at this as we would a toxin. That is nonsense. Electromagnetic fields are essential to the body throughout. We are operating with the wrong model, expecting that we will see a dose-response relationship. The appropriate model is more like a radio tuner. You can listen to some nice music when the signal that is transduced properly is tuned to the right frequency. But if you tune it wrong, you get static that can wreak havoc. I showed that I could take a beating heart within a frog and set it up so that I put out a very, very small signal, way below our safety standards today. If I put out a single pulse at different points in the cardiogram cycle, most of the time the heart ignored it. If I put it in at a certain point in the heart cycle, I could stop the heart by tuning it incorrectly."

Not surprisingly, the Web sites that the CTIA currently cites as saying that cell phones are safe do not reach those conclusions, which you can check by looking at links at www.devradavis.com. Similarly, the CTIA official statement that the peer-reviewed evidence shows that there is no evidence of increased risk and there is no known mechanism through which such a risk could happen represents a highly skewed reading of the literature.

In order to find any increased risk, you need two things. You need to study a lot of people and you need to be sure that they have been clearly exposed. This is how any analysis gets what is called power. In effect, the Interphone study lacked power for one main reason: Exposure in the study — defined as long and heavy use of cell phones — was neither high nor long. The project defined a cell phone user as someone who made one call a week for six months, and the average length of using a cell phone was less than six years. The well-pub-licized Danish study of several hundred thousand cell phone users actually included only two cases that had used a phone for a decade. In contrast, the Swedish team had a dozen long-term users with brain tumors, many more heavy users, and saw a significantly increased risk of brain tumors. And Interphone had less than one in ten of its cases with such regular use.

It is a matter of great concern that when you look at all the Interphone studies combined, without taking into account how long phones have been used, it looks as though cell phones actually protect users against brain tumors. But when you look at those few studies that included people who had used phones for a decade or more, the results show that heavy cell phone use causes brain tumors. If you consider all of the studies that have been published, most of them have not followed people for a decade. But if you examine only those studies that have analyzed people for a decade or longer you find one thing: Every single one of them shows that long-term heavy use of cell phones has increased the risks of brain tumors.

Still, using the language of science, the Interphone report concludes that we can't be sure whether the increased risks of brain tumors that they found is genuinely tied with cell phone use. "The possible effects of long-term heavy use of mobile phones require further investigation." In other words, more research is needed.

Indeed. The question is what are we supposed to do now

Public Health Isn't Just About Epidemiology Either

But wait a minute, at this stage of our scientific understanding of mice and men one has to ask, should how we treat cell phones depend on whether we already see evidence they have produced measurable increases in brain tumors in the general population? After all, the International Agency for Research on Cancer (part of the World Health Organization) and the European Environment Agency state as a matter of policy that any compound that causes cancer or other chronic illnesses in animals should be regarded as if it could cause such diseases in humans. If you take this preventive approach, then the matter of radio frequency radiation and health looks quite a bit different. Epidemiology is then seen not as the definitive resolution of the issue, but as only one piece of the puzzle that can be used to understand brain cancer or other chronic illnesses that may be tied with cell phone radiation. Another important component can and should come from experimental studies like those carried out by many of the researchers described in earlier chapters.

Once we begin to think about experimental findings, we are not limited to waiting for bodies to succumb to illnesses like brain cancer that we know can take decades to form. We can also look at conditions that arise more quickly and can be more easily studied in cell cultures and animals. Earlier we learned that cell phone radiation affects fast-growing sperm, but think about how such radiation might impact another vulnerable part of all mammalial bodies — our eyes.

The human eye includes several layers. The outermost cover includes a transparent, rounded cornea and an opaque, white sclera that shield the eye. The next layer contains the iris that gives us our dominant color, the small dark, round hole or pupil that allows light to enter the eyeball, and the ciliary body to which muscles are attached that allow us to focus. Behind the pupil and iris sits the transparent, elliptical, and somewhat flexible lens. Over time, we tend to lose that flexibility and with it the ability to focus as easily, which is why most of us need reading glasses once we hit the age of forty.

The lens of the eye occurs near the very front of the eyeball and should be clear as glass, allowing us to focus light onto the retina at the back of the eye, so that we can form images that get sent to the brain through the optic nerve. If the lens becomes cloudy and covered by opaque materials, we eventually lose the capacity to see completely. The first signs of a cataract can be blurriness and difficulty focusing. Eventually, if not surgically removed, cataracts can lead to complete blindness.

Cataracts of the eye, like brain tumors, can take decades to form in humans. In fact, cataracts are quite common as we age and those tied with growing older tend to form in both eyes at about the same time. More than half of us have some sign of cataract in both eyes if we reach the age of seventy. But electromagnetic radiation has the capacity to do something quite unusual both in humans and animals. After World War II, U.S. Navy veteran and Pearl Harbor survivor Milton M. Zaret became an ophthalmologist in Scarsdale, New York. He examined about sixteen hundred air force, navy, and army workers to see whether their jobs with radar and related radio frequency expo- sures had any impact on the fronts of their eyes. Typically, half of all people age seventy have cataracts in both their eyes. Almost no one should have cataracts in their twenties or thirties. And nobody should have a cataract in only one eye, unless something has damaged the membrane that normally protects our vision.

In the summer of 1961, at the height of the Cold War, just four years after the Soviets gained space superiority with the launch of Sputnik, Zaret was examining a group of civilian radar technicians in Thule, Greenland. He saw two men who would forever change his way of thinking about cataracts and microwaves. These fellows were under age thirty and had worked together ten days earlier, repairing what they had been told was a shut-down radar antenna. Electric sparks shot out of their metal screwdrivers. This meant only one thing: The antenna had in fact not been shut down but had been hot with power. Neither man reported feeling anything at all after this incident, as they set to work. This meant that the radio frequency from the antennas had not been strong enough to cause heat or pain to the eye. Still, they had each developed cataracts — something Zaret had never seen before in such young men. In other radar technicians, Zaret began to see a pattern, which was also evident to David Karr, former director of the National Laboratory at Los Alamos. Damage would occur in one eye — typically that used to focus the antennas — and the effect would be on the back surface of the lens, not on the front. Zaret was confident he had discovered that a "posterior cataract" was in fact uniquely tied with microwave exposure. By the end of the 1960s, Zaret had assembled more than three dozen cases of men with cataracts in only one eye at the back of the lens. All of them were under the age of forty. By 1972, no longer in the military, Zaret had published a theory in the *Transactions on Biomedical Engineering* that what lay behind all this eye damage could also account for a number of other problems that might arise from microwave-like radiation. Such radiation, he reasoned, affected the lining or membranes of the eye, the heart, the blood vessels, and perhaps even the brain.

The cardiovascular elastic membrane, like the lens capsule elastic membrane, is constantly under the stress of relative stretch and relaxation as it helps to sustain the hydraulic pressure of the circulatory system. . . . It is interesting to note that a gross parallel could be drawn between the increased incidence of coronary artery disease and myocardial infarction in urban centers and the increased ambient levels of electronic smog in these environments.

This research is one part of the puzzle that leads Dr. Hardell to conclude that Alan Marks's brain tumor was caused by cell phones. He takes what is known from observing those few people who have used phones heavily and over a long period and combines it with experimental studies, like those carried out by Allan Frey close to fifty years ago, or those completed more recently by Leif Salford and Henrietta Nittby in Sweden, or those published just this year by Lukas Margaritis and Adamantia Fragopoulou.

As Oprah's favorite doctor, the acclaimed cardiac surgeon and physician Dr. Mehmet Oz, declared, when looking at all the evidence together, "I've heard enough to make me rethink my cell phone use and that of my children."

When it comes to studying cell phones and brain tumors, how are we supposed to proceed? There can be no double blinding in studying the matter. It would be unethical to put people into experimental groups and deliberately expose some of them and not expose others and then wait to see whether the exposed group develops more brain tumors. So how is it ethical to have billions of young people use a technology whose dangers will only become broadly evident in forty years?

Medicine today is becoming a much more scientific discipline that relies on reproducible results to decide what drugs or surgeries work best to treat illness. One of the novel parts of health care reform is that it actually requires that many widely used medical procedures and medications be looked at carefully and not be used until and unless they have been shown to work. How do physicians go about figuring out what works in treating disease? Whenever they can do so, they rely on a gold standard of using a randomized clinical trial. Such a trial typically starts out with two comparable groups of people who have a given ailment, whether a torn anterior cruciate ligament or an abnormal heartbeat. After those who are affected have agreed to be part of a study, one group gets whatever is the standard treatment, while the other receives whatever novel intervention is being proposed. Sometimes, yet a third group is allowed to be given no treatment at all, just as a way to gauge the natural history of the problem. Yes, sometimes wounded knees and strange palpitations will go away on their own, so using a group that gets no treatment, or one that thinks it is getting a treatment but is not, is a way to test for what naturally happens over time.

In the past, medicine came by its preeminent reputation because most disease is really self-limiting. People do tend to heal on their own from a remarkable panoply of disorders if given the old treatment sometimes called tincture of time. Time is the one thing that every single being has less of as we get older. The mathematics are actually quite simple and follow the birthday anticipation rule. When you are three, a year is a third of your life and you wait what feels like eternity for your birthday, not really knowing what that is. When you are five, a year is one-fifth of your life and the wait for your birthday is marked by seasons that you have begun to understand do not take forever. When you are fifty, a year is 2 percent of your life and passes faster than you imagined it ever would. By the time you hit the age of some distinction in your sixties, where I am, birthdays start to pass by quickly, along with the friends and family whom you once could always count on.

With age, if we are fortunate, the proportion of our lives that we mark with any given period of time shrinks. It feels like a perpetuity waiting to be old enough to get a driver's license or to find out about college acceptance. But it feels like yesterday when we held our first grandchild, saw our own child graduate from college, or visited his first new home.

People who develop brain cancer, like those who deal with all other forms of this disease, develop a keen sense of staying in the right here and now. Time past, before the illness, lingers as memories of how it used to be, when bodies, minds, and hearts were taken for granted. Those whose brains have been invaded by foreign cells that know no limits tend to be frankly grateful for the chance the disease gives them to focus on the present.

My Unpublished Result

How does science figure out whether any external factor plays a role in causing cancer?

First of all we look at trends and ask if there has been any change in overall rates. It looks at first as if there's been no increase in brain tumors. But that turns out not to be the full story.

No doubt the total number of brain cancers is increasing because the population is growing larger and older. One way to look at patterns of brain cancer that take into account changes in the underlying population is to examine the number of cases that occur by creating a rate. We do this by adjusting for the number of people alive in any given age group. Thus in America and most industrial nations today, the rate of brain cancer is about fifty-seven per one hundred thousand people age seventy-five, and less than a tenth that of people under age twenty. The rate of glioma, the highly malignant tumor of the brain, in persons ages thirty to thirty-nine in the Interphone study looks a bit different: About one in every four cases of glioma in the Interphone report was diagnosed between the ages of thirty and forty.

In fact, my postdoctoral fellow Monica Han and I at Pittsburgh produced a series of analyses on rates of both benign and malignant brain tumors in Americans between the ages of twenty and forty from

1973 to 2005. Working with M.D. Anderson's Melissa Bondy and Ronald Herberman, then chief of The University of Pittsburgh Cancer Institute, we have shown that there is a real increase in both malignant gliomas and benign brain tumors in young adults. Our efforts to get this work published provide a case study in how hard it is to get tough news in print on this topic. I won't dwell on the details of this here—my peers have not yet reviewed this research, after all. Papers showing no increase in the overall brain cancer rate adjusted to the entire population have been published, while those taking a more sophisticated look at growing rates of brain tumors in young persons remain under review. Yet it is the young adults today who employ wireless technologies in ways that were impossible when the previous generation was in high school. Suffice it to say that we found that the number of people under age forty who can tell you just how horrible brain cancer is has been growing in the United States for the past three decades. We do not know why this is the case, merely that it is.

Waiting Until It Is Too Late

If new phones emit more radio frequency radiation and cell signals are absorbed into the brain, why, then, have most studies of human health, including the recent Interphone results, not found any problem?

Among the groups working on the Danish study was the International Epidemiology Institute (IEI), a group of seasoned, respected epidemiologists formerly employed by the National Cancer Institute. Paul Goldberg, editor of *The Cancer Letter*, told me that the IEI worked on the Danish Cancer Society study as "a business development opportunity." I wasn't sure what that meant. This group received no direct payment for its services. Now, that is an odd sort of business opportunity development. Or was it a kind of internship? Subsequently, the IEI has defended the cell phone industry in lawsuits filed by surviving family members of persons who died of brain tumors and were heavy cell phone users. So far, all of those cases have been won by the phone industry, arguing that proof of human harm has not been established. So, relax, there's no epidemic.

An interesting pattern of sponsorship of all this work has been depicted in a peer-reviewed paper in the National Institute of Environmental Health Sciences flagship journal, Environmental Health Perspectives. For the decade between 1995 and 2005, nearly all of the research sponsored by industry has found that cell phones are safe, while most of the studies independently funded have found a variety of problems. Henry Lai of the University of Washington has shown that the odds are very small that any industry-sponsored study will find that cell signals negatively impact health. This could be a coincidence, but Om Gandhi doesn't think so.

The prolonged drama and lack of results from the Interphone study have created what *The Economist* termed a "farrago of misinformation." Some of the study chiefs are no longer on speaking terms. They all agree that more research is needed. They do not agree on how to go about setting this up.

Dr. Hardell is not part of Interphone. But he is no longer a solo operator in finding that cell and cordless phones increase the risk of some brain tumors and a benign tumor of the hearing nerve called acoustic neuroma. Even the finally released Interphone results confirm Hardell: People who used phones the most for ten years or more have doubled risk of glioma. Most troubling are some reports from Hardell presented recently in London. Those who began using cell phones heavily as teenagers have four to five times more malignant brain tumors by their late twenties. For industry, whether in Canada or China, time postponed in having a product declared a problem means more money to be made. For those who have the luxury to think about public health, time spent waiting for more research can turn out to be profitable as well. Time usually gives us stronger information and clearer proof of harm — often in the form of more sickness and death — and incidentally can have the side benefit of providing more money for us and our students to do more research in the meantime.

No matter how hard I look at various ways researchers have tried to measure the incidence of brain cancer and its rate of change, I remain convinced we should not wait for proof that population-wide shifts have occurred before taking simple precautions to reduce direct exposure of our brains and bodies to cell phone radiation. Science on this complicated topic remains uncertain, for two reasons. First of all, science truly is complex and not easily understood by most of us. But a very large part of that uncertainty on this issue has been manufactured by those with deep pockets whose bottom line remains their primary focus. Many of those engaged in efforts to study cell phone radiation have, just as Gandhi said, made up their minds in advance. The fact that ready money has been there to support those who cast doubt on the dangers of radio frequency radiation certainly plays some role in the perpetuation of their views, as it did with tobacco, asbestos, benzene, and hormone replacement therapy.

The health of our children's and grandchildren's brains is not a matter that should be put on hold while we continue to debate technical matters. Certainly, the fact that the governments of Israel and France and Finland — to name just a few — are acting to reduce exposures to cell phone radiation and insisting on more public information should make us think hard about what we are doing. The existence of scientific conflict on this subject is in large part a reflection of the successful efforts of some to manufacture scientific doubt. In science, as in much of life, the perfect is the enemy of the pretty damn good. If we insist on seeing proof that an epidemic is already under way, before acting to restrain exposures to an agent that damages DNA, weakens the blood-brain barrier, and unleashes destructive free radicals throughout the body, we will condemn ourselves and our families to our lesser angels. There is no virtue in waiting until it is too late.

10

READING THE FINE PRINT

> *We can't always trust our common sense, and we don't always know good advice when we hear it, but if we work at it in a well-informed way, I think most of us can move at least a bit in that direction.*
> *~David H. Freedman*

For more than three centuries, the men and few women who work as actuaries have predicted the chances that various catastrophes will take place. If their calculations are right, insurance companies make money. If they are wrong, they can go broke. On some level insurance is the ultimate hedge — you pay a premium hoping that they get to keep it, because if whatever you are insuring against actually happens, then you will lose something big, perhaps even your home, your life, or your family members.

In the seventeenth century the self-made scientist-businessman John Graunt created the tools that eventually allowed people to understand just how to predict the occurrence of natural or humanmade disasters, whether from smoke and fires or floods. I wrote about him ten years ago and his relevance still hits me about once a week. Graunt was a master of assembling and making sense of ordinary information. He laid the foundation for the ways of categorizing, counting, and rendering facts and figures that would later change the way people thought about the connections between health and the surrounding world. In 1662, Graunt published a short book, *Natural and Political Observations Made Upon the Bills of Mortality*, that summed up his years of sorting and analyzing who died, where, when, and how.

He intended his work to provide the government and church with a rational way of setting policy, whether that required counting the number of fit fighting men or new surviving babies.

Graunt counted and organized people by sex, state, age, religion, trade, rank, degree, and how and where they died and what sickened them. In his system, deaths by "cancer, dog bytes, drowning, plague, fryght, childbirth, feaver, head-mould, rupture, scurvy, spotted feaver, stone, stopping of the stomach, stangury, teeth, ulcer, wormes, French pox [the British term for syphilis], small pox, and burnt in his bed" were recorded weekly. He reported on christenings and burials of males and females.

Whether Graunt ever profited from his tabulations is not clear. His little book went through at least five editions. It showed that it was possible to calculate, on the basis of a few facts about a person's life, how long and well they would live and the likelihood that they would die of a given disease. Graunt even allowed that the "prevalence of acute and epidemical diseases might give a measure of the state, and disposition of this Climate, and Air . . . as well as its food." The information assembled by Graunt and others became the basis for one of the earliest and soundest systems of true social security. Cities in England and elsewhere began to finance basic services through the sale of life annuities. At a time when the average person lived to age thirty-five, selling people the chance that they would collect money after age forty was such a sure thing that governments bet their funding on it. The Dutch began depending on such a system about the same time, with many towns staking their revenues on annuities sold. In London, you could buy insurance against numerous fates, from death by horse to loss of virginity.

The insurance industry was born. Large sums of money were moved around. Lawyers, of course, soon got in on the action. The language of all those warning labels you see on products you buy are written by groups of lawyers at the behest of insurance companies. Everybody wants to cut his losses and hedge his bets.

Hedging

Nowadays governments in most countries provide some sort of health insurance for many, if not all, of their citizens. Some of us have secondary insurance as well that kicks in when the first policy runs out. In the global world of indemnity, Swiss Re is the largest secondary insurance firm in the world. It handicaps huge firms and provides the ultimate backup when and if costs of any horrific event exceed the primary coverage. With 15,000 insured lives and costs of just twenty-six billion dollars from 133 natural catastrophes and 155 human-made disasters, 2009 was a very good year for the secondary insurance business; losses were quite low. In contrast, 2010 started off with a heavy hit, winter storm Xynthia in Europe and the earthquakes in Chile, Haiti, and Tibet. Then there was the volcanic eruption in Iceland that disrupted flights to and from Europe. Costs could easily run three times those of the year before.

About a decade ago, those who decide whether to offer secondary insurance to firms in Austria figured out they needed to know whether to provide protection against possible cell phone damages. That's why the Austrian government gave Professor Wilhelm Mosgoeller hundreds of thousands of euros to study how living cells respond to cell phone radiation from both 2G and the then newer 3G signals.

Mosgoeller conducted several different studies — all aimed at clarifying whether cell-phone-like signals had any impact. Working with human volunteers, his team measured their brain waves, how quickly they responded, and how well they remembered various things before and after they were exposed to typical cell phone signals for periods of five minutes to an hour. The participants in this study sat in comfortable chairs with cell-phone-like devices snuggled against their heads and had no way of knowing whether these devices were sending signals or doing nothing at all. Those analyzing the records of brain waves and speeds of response did not know whether the person they were studying had been exposed to true cell phone signals — so there was no way the observers could bias their results. When the codes for this study were broken they showed that persons exposed to cell phone signals had much faster responses when tested. But cell phone users also made more mistakes.

Another set of studies the Mosgoeller team produced examined human cells that can be kept alive in the laboratory, working with machines that issued precise radio frequency signals like those of modern phones. The machines were on for five minutes, off for ten minutes, for eight hours a day. Such exposures had no impact on the immune function of exposed cells. But a number of other abnormalities of the blood doubled or quadrupled in the cells that had received cell-phone-like exposure. This work was carried out under stringent controls that followed the highest standards of good laboratory practices. The findings of altered cell growth were repeated by several different laboratories working independently, with those evaluating the data having no idea which cells had and had not been exposed.

When his results were in, the Austrian workers' compensation system began paying workers for job-related health damages tied with cell phones. The insurance industry stopped writing policies to provide backup to the cell phone manufacturers. It deduced that while the risk of health damage from cell phones was not firmly established, there was enough troubling and well-documented evidence that cell phone signals do increase some measures of damage that it declines to take that risk on at all.

The Austrian insurance industry is not the only group to decide not to provide secondary insurance to cover cell phones. In 1999, John Fenn, an underwriter with one of the world's largest secondary insurers, the Stirling Group of Lloyd's of London, refused to insure cell phone manufacturers against health-related claims. Lloyd's writes policies on everything from Madonna's dancing to aircraft engines. In deciding not to insure coverage for future health problems tied with cell phones, the firm was responding to fears about cell phones, but also to growing scientific reports linking health risks to the brain and body with frequent cell phone use.

Newspaper accounts in *The Guardian, The Independent, The Mail, The Sun, The Telegraph,* and television reports on the BBC had tracked the deliberations of a committee chaired by the eminent British physician Sir William Stewart, which was reviewing evidence on health issues and cell phones. They learned that the Stewart Commission was about to release a report recommending limits on cell phone use and advising that children under age sixteen not use cell phones at all. The information was enough to convince the Stirling Group to stop providing secondary insurance to cell phone manufacturers.

Fenn explained, "There are people in the insurance market who close their eyes to the issue because they say there is no scientific proof of a problem. If you go back to asbestos, it 'wasn't a problem' at one time either."

Asbestos claims nearly destroyed Lloyd's in the early 1990s. The analogy with asbestos may be especially apt. The history of the failure to address asbestos risks is fraught with instances where industry manufactured doubt, undermined science, and manipulated government in order to extend its financial gain. Eventually, government found ways to regulate the asbestos industry, driven in large part by lawsuits that documented the long-standing duplicity of industry. Good government, good laws, reasonable negotiation can find ways to manage hazards like those that may stem from cell phone radiation. Whether it will take the press of lawsuits to get us there remains to be seen.

For Maine's Sake

In the state of Maine, depending on what part of the state a person hails from, he or she may be called a Mainer, a Mainah, or a Maniac. Andrea Boland is a legislator in Maine's statehouse who combines the state's famed independence of spirit with a principled conviction that just because nobody has ever tried to do a particular thing doesn't mean it shouldn't be done. Widowed, with two adult children, Boland first heard about the risks that cell phones pose for health when we met in Boston at a conference in 2007. In talking with her then about the final chapters of my book *The Secret History of the War on Cancer*, I had discussed cell phones as being one of the most troubling modern issues.

"We don't really know that today's cell phones are safe, despite the fact that more than half of all adults are using them, as are growing numbers of young children," I said. "I can't tell you if cell phones are dangerous, but I have lots of good reasons for concerns that they may be. I can tell you that the experimental evidence is deeply troubling. The absence of definitive human health consequences of cell phones now is not surprising. We really need to understand why other nations are acting to restrict their use and issuing warnings about their potential hazards."

Over the past three years, Boland has been talking privately about some puzzling issues: Why had the FDA decided that microwave ovens needed to be tested for safety when they were first marketed as radar ranges, because they cooked things and generated heat, but that cell phones — which operated with less power but at the same wavelength as microwave ovens — did not require any testing at all? Why had so many nations decided to advise that children not use cell phones and that adults take simple steps to reduce direct exposures to their heads and bodies? Why was there no American research under way on cell phone safety or impacts?

Boland has become well informed on the topic. She has an advisor from the cell phone industry and the Defense Department who insists on remaining anonymous. This fellow came forward when he heard of Boland's interest, because he had grown disgusted with the misrepresentations of science that he knew from the inside out because he had worked on building sophisticated electronic systems for years. He talks in the rapid speech of the supernerd/gifted child he once was. He is not surprised that laboratory results show increased damage to DNA from pulsed cell phone radiation. At the Maine hearings that he drove to attend, this anonymous Defense Department researcher told me why the idea that radio frequency radiation must be benign because you cannot feel heat from it right away is simply nonsense. He explained that there are superhot effects called supra-thermal effects that occur in very tiny spaces that are exposed to radio frequency radiation — hotspots.

"What it means to be thermal is that there is a distribution of speeds and motions among the molecules, so that the average energy in a small group is in equilibrium, kind of like a bunch of cars going sixty miles per hour northbound, and another bunch going southbound at the same speed. Their energy is calculated as half of their mass multiplied by velocity squared. When this distribution becomes stable, that's the thermal condition, with the energy being the same. Suprathermal is where you would find a bunch of cars going well above the average speed, and there is not enough time for the smoothing down of the speed, so bonds are breaking before things have a chance to cool down and distribute overall.

"We could use machine guns to heat our rooms, it would work, it would just be hazardous. The heat energy from the bullets would spread out over time, but all the mess would not be helpful. If ionic conductivity decreased with temperature, we would not be seeing effects such as single and double strand breaks. We are seeing such damage because heat is occurring in the tiniest spaces that cannot be picked up by our current systems of measurement."

"So," I asked, "what do you think of the idea that we should make all cell phones comply with international averaging standards that use ten grams of tissue as opposed to one gram?"

He replied with the cynical smirk and sardonic tone of someone who spends most of his time in the laboratory. "Of course, international compatibility is a good idea, but they are going about it backwards. If what you are trying to do is get the most radiation into our heads and allow the most hotspots to form, then the ten gram standard is the way to go because of course you will have lots of tiny areas with humongous heat and most of the areas will have none. But that's not how I want to treat my own brain."

Boland is not taking on the international standards issue directly, hoping that sensible minds will prevail. For now, she is focusing on how people use their phones today. She and I discussed the hearings convened by U.S. Congressman Dennis Kucinich, as chair of the Domestic Policy Subcommittee of the Committee on Oversight and Government Reform, in July 2008. We talked about the snub industry gave those hearings, which were held during the last months of the George W. Bush administration. The Cellular Telecommunications Industry Association (CTIA) officially said that it would let the science speak for itself on the subject and refused to attend.

A CTIA spokesperson said the organization's lack of testimony at the Kucinich hearing shouldn't be seen as a dodge.

At the 2008 hearing, Dr. Ronald B. Herberman, a distinguished cancer biologist and my former boss, explained what made him decide to issue a warning to the more than three thousand staff members of the University of Pittsburgh Cancer Institute. He had seen enough scientific studies on the topic — produced mostly by experts outside of the United States — to know that holding a microwavelike signaling device next to the brain did not make sense. His advice to the staff was simple: Don't use a phone next to your head. Use a speakerphone or earpiece and restrict children's use.

Herberman explained his reasoning. "I cannot tell this committee that cell phones are definitely dangerous but I certainly cannot tell you that they are safe." One big part of the problem is that most studies have been done for too short a period of time to find any increased risk of brain tumors. Testifying at this same hearing, Dr. David Carpenter, epidemiologist and former dean of the School of Public Health at the University at Albany, mentioned that the study by Swedish physician researcher Lennart Hardell had found an association between prolonged cell phone use and two types of brain cancers — with those who had begun using a cell phone before age twenty having five times more brain tumors than those who had not. Kucinich asked whether the evidence was sufficient that "there should be national standards of warning or precaution relating to the use of cell phones for children?"

Both Carpenter and Herberman agreed.

Carpenter added this warning: "I think evidence is certainly strong enough for warnings that children should not use cell phones. I think failure to do that is going to lead us to an epidemic of brain cancer in the future."

Boland knows that many other experts and nations have issued similar advice, including physician and writer David Servan-Schreiber (who kindly wrote the foreword to this book) and Elmer Huerta,

M.D., then president of the American Cancer Society, who translated Herberman's advisory in his Spanish-language broadcasts and blogs throughout Latin America. She also has read much of the comprehensive review of the literature provided by the BioInitiative Report organized by Carpenter and Cindy Sage, an expert consultant on electromagnetic field evaluation and reduction who has spearheaded much public discussion on the issue.

By the fall of 2009, Washington, D.C., had a new president and a new set of priorities. A call to testify before Congress could no longer be so comfortably ducked. Environmental Health Trust, the nonprofit public charity I set up, convened an expert conference on cell phones and health, with participants from ten nations and support from the U.S. National Institute of Environmental Health Sciences, Carolyn Fine Friedman and the Milton Friedman Foundation, the International Commission on Electromagnetic Safety, and private donors. (My Web site includes papers, slides, and videos from this important meeting.) When Senators Arlen Specter of Pennsylvania and Tom Harkin of Iowa convened a hearing on the subject of cell phones and health, September 14, 2009, the CTIA sent Linda Erdreich, an epidemiologist who had worked for a number of different industries and published extensively in some of the top ranked journals in the field. For the CTIA, Erdreich had played a decisive role extensively reviewing and reshaping the work of the young researcher Joshua Muscat, originally produced for the Wireless Technology Research (WTR) program headed up by George Carlo — as noted in the previous chapter. Early drafts of Muscat's small study that were presented to scientific conferences showed a tripled risk of brain tumor with cell phone use. After Erdreich's interventions, by the time any results appeared in print, that risk had disappeared.

Erdreich testified that most studies on the topic of brain cancer and cell phones had been negative. She did not address the facts that many of those studies are funded by the industry; most of them have studied people for less than ten years when phones were not used as they are now for hours a day; and none of them has studied children or young adults. In the long awaited and officially inconclusive Interphone study the average user spoke on a phone for two hours a month — something many young people now do every day. Senator Specter had more than the usual interest in the topic, as a brain tumor survivor himself. When the senator asked Erdreich whether she could say with certainty that there was no harmful effect of cell phone radiation on the health of individuals, Erdreich said, quite reasonably, that no science can say definitively that there are no harmful effects. She did not mention the evidence of harmful effects from researchers like Frey, Gandhi, Adlkofer, and Mosgoeller, nor the fact that every study that has been able to look at people who have been big talkers on cell phones for a decade or more has found increased risks of brain tumors.

Siegal Sadetzki is a highly respected epidemiologist and physician who drafted the Israeli government's official warning on cell phones and is a leader of the Interphone analysis. Israel is only now implementing a clean air act and tends to be quite reserved regarding matters of environmental protection. The nation also has a very sophisticated appreciation of radar and other microwave-based technology, which so far have provided it with some valuable protection. Sadetzki explained that while she was not certain cell phone radiation caused brain tumors, she had ample reasons for concern. Among those reasons was her own work showing that heavier cell phone users in Israel developed significantly more tumors of the cheek — the parotid gland — than those who did not use cell phones. Other reports commissioned by the Israel Dental Association found two troubling results: Since 2003, rates of this cheek tumor have tripled. Lately more than one of every four cases of parotid gland tumors occurs in someone under the age of twenty. Today Israelis often do not have landlines and are among the highest users of cell phones in the world — more than half of them talk an hour a day.

An intense, attractive Israeli woman, Sadetzki acknowledged that she was personally troubled by what she had learned, even though there was a need for more study. Those studies that have followed people who have used phones heavily for a decade or longer, like her own work finding doubled rates of tumors in the cheek, do find increased risks of brain tumors. As a public health official she has seen enough red flags to justify public warnings.

As Sadetzki said, "It is far better to prevent harm using simple and low-cost measures than to wait for long-term results to confirm a health hazard that has already occurred," she said. "Therefore we must be prepared to act before scientific certainty has been achieved."

At the same Environmental Health Trust conference Michael Thun, senior vice president of the American Cancer Society, reported his view that when looking at all the published studies to date the data on brain tumor risk so far had been reassuring.

"Reassuring? Reassuring? How can you say such a thing!" Sadetzki asked in astonishment. "Look, we are not certain that cell phones increase brain tumor risk, we agree on that. But there are lots of reasons for concerns at this point."

To his credit, Thun agreed. He has since told *Parade* magazine that while studies on brain tumors and cell phones as a whole do not show an increased risk, three recent studies do find increased risks of malignant glioma. He also allowed that "if cell phones were harmful, then it is conceivable that children might be more vulnerable."

Officially, the American Cancer Society agrees with the U.S. government Web sites: More data are needed. But it is reasonable to ask, where are those data going to come from? Who's going to pay for them? Who's going to gather them?

In questioning what could be done now, Senator Harkin held up his own wired headset. All those testifying except Erdreich indicated that they used such devices as a way to reduce direct exposure to their brains. Both Senators Specter and Harkin were surprised to learn that cell phone manuals include fine print advice about holding phones away from the body, even though these warnings do not appear any-where on the phones themselves. "Does anybody know why or when this advice started to be given out?" he wondered.

About as many people read the fine print legalese on paperwork that comes in the package with a new cell phone as read their credit card agreements or warnings with prescription drugs. Indeed, the language has similar formalities. If we are going to overcome the disconnect between the public perception of harmless cell phones and what researchers have found, we are going to have to get beyond that tiny print and obfuscating language.

A Plain Warning

As of spring 2010, the Motorola V195 includes a warning to keep the phone one inch from the user's body; the BlackBerry 8300, 1.98 of an inch; the Nokia 1100, one-fourth of an inch; and the iPhone, five-eighths of an inch. The HTC Droid Eris cell phone from Verizon contains a "Product Safety and Warranty Information" booklet. On page 11 it is recommended "that no part of the human body be allowed to come too close to the antenna during operation of the equipment." A customer query about this was referred to an online appendix, which explained on page 219: "To comply with RF exposure requirements, a minimum separation distance of 1.5 cm must be maintained between the user's body and the handset, including the antenna." These and other advisories can be found on my Web site in the small print in which they occur and can be magnified by clicking on an icon. A reader might think it was just a matter of complying with a silly rule that government had produced.

In arguing for her bill Boland figured she would call everyone's bluff. She knew enough about the history of empty promises and the use of science as a justification for inaction.

In arguing for her bill, Boland proposed that a specific warning label be placed on phones in the state of Maine and got a bill to do so before a committee of the legislature. The proposed warning label would read: "This device emits electromagnetic radiation, exposure to which may cause brain cancer. Users, especially pregnant women and children, should keep away from the head and body." Neither she nor anyone else thinks a warning like this will result in the collapse of the cell phone industry. It would simply promote safer cell phones. Companies might advertise how much safer their cell phones were — not unlike, say, the more efficient refrigerators and washing machines tagged with the Energy Star. The result would be less cell phone radiation getting into our bodies, not the end of cell phone civilization.

Boland brought Gandhi and Adlkofer, and some of the world's leading scientists to Augusta, Maine, in March 2010, where they provided concise summaries of the science. Not about to be out-maneuvered by a lone citizen-legislator, the CTIA was there in full force some three months earlier, having hired some of the state's top Democrat and Republican lobbyists. One savvy professional regis-tered consumer lobbyist of Maine was called in by some of the big firms and told that if he ever expected to get other work in this state, he should stay out of this issue. Mindy Brown testified, describing Coach Dan Brown's struggles with brain cancer before his death. Ellie and Alan Marks soberly depicted the agonizing challenges of Alan's brain tumor. Mindy and Dan Brown's son Larry held up a copy of the six point type, very small print that reads, "Warning, do not hold the phone on the body."

When Dane Snowden, vice president for external and state affairs of the CTIA, was asked by Representative Peter Stuckey to explain why cell phone manuals included such warnings today, he replied he would have to get back to the committee. Snowden certainly has experience with consumer matters, having previously served as chief of the Consumer and Governmental Affairs Bureau of the Federal Communications Commission. The FCC has never had a health expert on its staff. But its recent postings on this issue have taken a precautionary turn, telling people that if they want to reduce exposure there are simple ways to do so by using headsets and speakerphones and not keeping the phone on the body.

An especially strange presentation was made by Dora Mills, M.D., head of the Centers for Disease Control and Prevention of the state of Maine. Dr. Mills spent much of the hearing outside signaling that she had more important matters to do than sit through what international experts had to say on the issue. She did not listen to the testimonies of the brain tumor victims. For the record, she provided a highly selective reading of a pamphlet from the UK government, which she handed out. The fact that she did this suggests that Dr. Mills was betting that most of those on the committee would not take the time to read what she had given them but would rely on her to have provided the gist of it. Dr. Mills did not do this. Instead, she read just one sentence: "The balance of current research evidence suggests that exposures to radio waves below levels set out in international guidelines do not cause health problems for the general population."

But she did not read the next sentences:

"However, there is some evidence that changes in brain activity can occur below these guidelines, but it isn't clear why. There are significant gaps in our scientific knowledge.

"This has led a group of independent experts — commissioned by the Government . . . to recommend a "precautionary approach" to the use of mobile phones until more research findings become available.

"If you use a mobile phone, you can choose to minimize your exposure to radio waves. These are ways to do so:

- Keep your calls short
- Consider relative SAR values when buying a new phone."

Nor did she read this recommendation from the same pamphlet: "The widespread use of mobile phones by children (under the age of 16) should be discouraged for non-essential calls."

Dr. Mill's selective reading could provide a riff for the comedian Stephen Colbert railing against blindly following "sheeple." In any case, I hope that when the Maine legislature next considers this issue, the harried citizen-legislators will have had the time to review the pamphlet, the extensive submitted testimony (that can be found on the Web site), and even this book. Several citizens from Maine spoke in support, including local physician Meryl Nass; Michael Belliveau, head of the state's Environmental Health Strategy Center; Pamela Gerry, public health nurse and National Health Federation board member; Jody Spear, activist and consumer advocate; and Elisa Boxer-Cook, who spoke movingly about concerns for her young children.

As the public hearing wound down, a retired emergency room physician, Paul Leibow, rose. He said he had originally attended the briefing out of curiosity. But he felt compelled to speak, both as a citizen and as a physician who had seen so many puzzling cases of brain cancer recently.

"This is stunning new information to me and to most of us. We need to pay attention here."

Ken Carr of Woolwich, Maine, called the bill silly, but did not mention his own work for the industry and investments in wireless technology. Opposition predictably came from the CTIA representatives. Democrat governor John Baldacci, who has spearheaded wireless and broadband development across the state, opposed the bill and never read any of the expert testimony. In April 2010, the state of Maine announced expansion of its ties with Verizon, Time Warner, and other Internet service providers, by launching a program to expand state access called Connect ME — connect Maine. The governor did not have time to meet with the international experts. He may have confused their concerns about promoting safer cell phone use with a general antitechnology stance.

Ellie Marks told me, "Dr. Mills's speech parroted industry statements. She said if we put a label on cell phones we will need to label everything from apples to xylophones. She also commented how she could walk across the room, have a ceiling tile fall on her head, and kill her, so perhaps we need a warning on the tiles."

This is not the stuff of serious, reasonable discussion.

Ellie is angry, and who can blame her? She continued, "One representative actually said even though she has friends that have died from brain tumors that she thinks was from their cell phone use, she feels the consumer should use common sense. No one on that committee ever said that it was the duty of the government or industry to prove that phones were safe in the first place! We pay taxes so our government can better protect and serve us."

So far, no one has got back to the Maine committee or to Senators Specter or Harkin explaining why industry is inserting fine print warnings inside packaging that few people see, but refusing to put warnings directly on phones. When I brought this to their attention in the spring of 2010, senior staff of the FDA and FCC appeared surprised to see that these warnings appear with all new smart phones.

Boland holds that "industry is doing the least they can. They are printing the tiniest notices buried deep within manuals in packaging that nobody keeps. All this does is bring the phone to a point where it just barely passes the standard emission allowed for large men and cannot protect children, pregnant women, and the rest of us."

About Those Standards Again

Robert C. Kane was a Motorola engineer for thirty years. On March 2, 1993, he received United States of America Patent and Trademark Office patent number 5191217 for a method and apparatus for field emission device electrostatic electron beam focusing. This was one of about two dozen different critical patents Kane and his colleagues held for improving the operations of cell phones, displays, connections, and efficiency.

Kane was a hands-on engineer. At Motorola for more than two decades, Robert C. Kane was part of the proud team that tested the first phones and made sure that they actually worked. In the old days Motorola did not use robots to test phones, it used engineers. Kane was often volunteered into testing devices, holding them next to his head for hours while signal strength and sound clarity were adjusted.

By 1997, Kane's interest had become intensely personal. He had developed two primary brain tumors and become convinced that all his work as a human test subject on phones had caused his illness. He began to plow through old records of biological testing in animals and cell cultures. What he found out shocked him. He became persuaded that using a cell phone had become a form of Russian roulette. In 2001, he self-published Cellular Telephone Russian Roulette. This book cannot be found in bookstores today. The best I could come up with was a few old copies offered for more than a hundred dollars each.

At one point when he was already ill, Kane contacted Om Gandhi, the former Motorola consultant and professor of engineering, to ask for his help in understanding how much microwave radiation he had been exposed to. Gandhi remembers meeting Kane in a hallway outside a professional meeting of the Bioelectromagnetics Society in Copenhagen.

"Kane said to me, 'I'm dying of a brain tumor, what can you tell me about what I was exposed to?' at the meeting in Copenhagen.

Soon after I had finished talking to Kane, the industry folks came to my room and knocked on my door. These were guys I knew then. They had been watching me talking to this fellow and I had not realized how dishonest they all were at the time. They told me, 'You don't want to talk to him, because he's a troublemaker.'"

I asked Gandhi what he thought about Kane's ideas now and he grew quiet.

"Look, I guess I was naïve. I had worked with industry for years. I trusted these folks. I really wanted to believe that these were good guys and for a while I think some of them were. But not anymore. What they have done with the standards today is a travesty."

For decades, Gandhi was on all of the original committees that developed models to set the standards for radio frequency devices, even before cell phones existed. He knows how to build these models from the bottom up and from the inside out. He understands in ways that few others can all of the strengths and limits of models of the brain.

Typically reserved, Gandhi has become sufficiently outraged that he has agreed to spend some time talking with activists seeking to require warnings on cell phones, and he has shared detailed information about formerly secret formulae that he devised for calculating safety limits for phones.

"Basically, the formula that we created to estimate the safe specific absorption rate for humans rested on finding out the level at which animals would stop working for food rewards. One can ask now whether that appears to be the best way to proceed, but that is what we did then. But there has been lots of monkeying around with our work. You see, we figured that people would hold phones right next to their ear. But lately industry has played around with that assumption, and all of the models put the test phone almost a half an inch from the ear. This seems like a small distance, but for microwave radiation and for the even lower electromagnetic radiation from the phone, it's enormous. This is because the strength of the signal falls off with the cube or even to the fourth power of the near distance from the brain. From what I can tell, new phones today tested with this artificial spacer actually allow four times more exposure to get into the brains of our children.

"Frankly the idea that ICNIRP is pushing that we should basically increase exposures and set standards based on how much radiation enters ten grams of tissue rather than one gram is preposterous. Of course, it would be good for the world to have one set of standards. But if we use the ten gram approach, we will dramatically increase the amount that can get into much smaller and still developing areas of the brains of our children.

"This is wrong and it needs to stop."

In the middle of a winter storm, Gandhi flew from Salt Lake City to Boston and took the train to Portland and then drove to Augusta to present his views to the Maine legislature.

The Golden Gate Opens

In June 2010, Mayor Gavin Newsom and commissioners of San Francisco — concerned that most people have no idea that cell phones release radio frequency radiation — offered city legislation affirming that the public has two basic rights: the right to know that cell phones release radio frequency radiation and the right to be able to read information about how to reduce exposures, rather than unearth warnings from tiny print in packaging materials that most of us discard. The CTIA countered this proposal. They argued that the public would be confused by making this information simpler to find and could erroneously conclude that some phones were safer than others. In opposing Mayor Newsom's proposal, the CTIA issued a full-page color ad in the Sunday *xw* on June 7, 2010, featuring a happily talking health care professional holding a cell phone closer to her head than the manufacturers advise and boldly declaring that cell phones have not been linked with brain cancer. Yet.

Scientific uncertainties, while indisputable, in this instance did not become the excuse for doing nothing. Environmental Health Trust board and staff members Harry V. Lehmann and Ellie Marks met with city supervisors and staff, as did Renee Sharp with the Environmental Working Group. Recapping her impassioned testimony to the U.S. Congress and the Maine legislature, Marks provided a riveting case — her husband Alan's brain tumor might have been avoided if anyone had told him about the need to keep cell phone radiation away from the brain. Lehmann, an experienced litigator with training in engineering, wrote to each supervisor and the mayor about the growing science behind the case for precaution, explaining that he had lost his two closest middle-age associates to brain tumors. Each of them, like Ellie's husband, Alan Marks, had been first adopters of cell phones.

When the bill was signed, the CTIA issued a press statement the next day, June 22, 2010, announcing that they would no longer hold their annual meetings worth almost eighty million dollars in revenue in this technological Mecca.

"CTIA and the wireless industry are disappointed that the San Francisco Board of Supervisors has approved the so-called "Cell Phone Right-to-Know" ordinance. Rather than inform, the ordinance will potentially mislead consumers with point of sale requirements suggesting that some phones are "safer" than others based on radio frequency (RF) emissions. In fact, all phones sold legally in the U.S. must comply with the Federal Communications Commission's safety standards for RF emissions. According to the FCC, all such compliant phones are safe phones as measured by these standards. The scientific evidence does not support point of sale requirements that would suggest some compliant phones are "safer" than other compliant phones based on RF emissions.

While we have enjoyed bringing our three day fall show to San Francisco five times in the last seven years, which has meant we've brought more than 68,000 exhibitors and attendees and had an economic impact of almost $80 million to the Bay Area economy, the Board of Supervisors' action has led us to decide to relocate our show. We are disappointed to announce that the 2010 CTIA Enterprise and Applications show in October will be the last one we have in San Francisco for the foreseeable future. We have already been contacted by several other cities that are eager to work with us and understand the tremendous benefits that wireless technology and our show can provide their area."

In their private lobbying against the bill, the CTIA had raised this threat with the city. One city official privy to the negotiations said, "The Mayor had always said that his city was not for sale and it's not. The law goes into effect in February 2011, along with a major public education campaign for retailers and the public."

11

THE WORLD FROM NOW ON

The right to search for truth implies also a duty.

~Albert Einstein

T he short history of public unease about cell phones provides an instructive pattern. Each time anyone raises the prospect that cell phones could prove harmful, and manages to get some media attention, whether through the publication of a new experimental finding, the filing of a lawsuit, the conduct of a state or congressional hearing, or the publication of some sassy magazine story about passionate activists, the response is the same. Industry agrees that this could be a problem and calls for and begins what looks like a major program of research.

In 1993, as the first lawsuits were filed alleging that cell phones improbably caused Susan Reynard's brain tumor, the well-funded twenty-eight-million-dollar, six-year program of research called the Wireless Technology Research (WTR) initiative, run by George Carlo, was set up ostensibly to produce an important independent body of research on the human and experimental impacts of radio frequency radiation. The WTR produced two volumes of research that were presented to symposiums held in Rome, Italy, and Long Beach, California, in 1995 and 1997. These can be purchased from an online retailer for $279.

When it comes to the lingua franca of science — the peer-reviewed journal article — the WTR directly produced no major publications. Perhaps this failure to publish peer-reviewed results was what was intended all along, as Louis Slesin of *Microwave News* alleges. Perhaps the failure came about because twenty-eight million dollars just was not enough to get the job done, as Carlo claims. Whatever the truth of the matter, the fact is that this large program ate up a decade, millions of dollars, and led to no change in policy.

Today's standards for cell phones were set in 1993, based on models that used a very large heavy man with an eleven-pound head talking for six minutes, when fewer than 10 percent of all adults had cell phones. Half of all ten-year-olds now have cell phones. Some young adults use phones for more than four hours a day; schools are providing textbooks through them and textbook publishers know this channel is a booming business. However many hours our children may be using cell phones close to their bodies every day, their brains and gonads will be exposed to levels of radio frequency that were set for this long-ago, big, quiet blockhead.

In 1997 and 2000, when questions about the potential health impacts of cell phones were raised at congressional hearings by Congressman Edward Markey and Senator Joseph Lieberman, respectively, the General Accounting Office duly issued two separate reports. Each said the same thing: More research was needed.

The call for research becomes a sop to delay doing anything except appearing to study a problem. This call for more investigations remains the one thing about which all parties are agreed — including officials in the states of Maine and California as well as the CTIA,

Congressional Representatives Kucinich, Markey, and Carolyn Malo-
ney, and Senators Harkin and Specter.

A superficial reading of what is termed the preponderance of the
evidence shows that cell phone radiation has little biological impact.
So, are those concerned about cell phones merely Luddites full of
apprehension about the modern world? That would be the case if
science proceeded simply like democracy, where the candidate with
the most votes wins. But as we have seen throughout this book, not all
scientific studies should be accorded equal weight. Where you stand
on this issue often depends on who paid for the chair you sit on. So
many studies show no impact of radio frequency radiation on our
bodies because of three distinct factors.

First, in previous decades military and industrial interests have
sometimes simply terminated research suggesting that cell phone
radiation may be harmful. Second, more recently, they have commissioned scientists to develop critiques of findings they do not like
and even to come up with what are purported to be studies aimed at
replicating cell phone dangers that actually do not repeat the original
work, but look enough like they do to raise doubts. One longtime
federal expert in the field explains the routine,

"If you want to undermine a study, you hire another scientist who
is new to the field and have him carry out research that looks very
close to the result you do not like. Only in some critical and fundamental ways this supposed replication is different. You change five
things from the original experiment. Maybe the cell line is one that
you happen to know will not respond to microwave energy, and the
exposure is continuous rather than pulsed. Then the results come and
lo and behold! You have findings that do not repeat the previous work.
Scientists do not like to be outliers. They follow the crowd."

So long as people are in doubt, things continue as they are. This
process of doubt production effectively discredits both the science

and the scientists working in the field of radio frequency radiation and health. That is why one colleague who left the field says that "working on radio frequency radiation has become the third rail — you touch it and you die."

Third, among scientists themselves, there is a powerful force creating what effectively becomes an insidious form of self-censorship.

Dariusz Leszczynski has the personal intensity of a man who would rather spend most of his waking hours thinking about basic scientific questions than sail or hike around his beautiful homeland in Finland. He has two doctoral degrees in the sciences. Leszczynski has been one of four research professors in Finland's national Radiation and Nuclear Safety Authority for more than two decades. He has served as a visiting professor at Harvard Medical School and currently is the Guangbiao Professor in the bioelectromagnetics laboratory of the medical school in Hangzhou, China. His research probing the ways that living cells respond to radio frequency radiation like that emitted by modern cell phones is supported by national authorities in many countries and by industry and private foundations.

In talking about why so many of his colleagues have participated in studies that become a form of self-censorship designed to raise doubt and produce little clear evidence, Leszczynski is philosophical.

"Scientists need the money to support research and their students. If the conclusion of a given scientific study is not in line with sponsors' expectations that no health effect will be found, that work is not likely to get additional funding. So, some scientists might be tempted to exercise a form of self-censorship and downplay the significance of their own work in order to not lose support."

In 2002, Leszczynski produced an elegant finding that might have been a turning point in the history of cell phones. He showed that after just one hour of exposure to pulsed cell phone signals like those we get from ordinary phones today, endothelial cells from the blood looked different. The reason this finding was such a bombshell was that the work came from the government laboratory in Finland. Leszczynski's research supported results produced years earlier by Frey in the 1970s and later by Salford in the early 1990s, showing that low levels of cell-phone-like exposure may impact the blood-brain barrier. Using the measured cadences of a scientist, Leszczynski said that if this same change in endothelial cells occurred in real people, it meant that molecules that could damage brain cells could enter the brain. But perhaps humans have some protection against this in real life?

In the mantra of science, Leszczynski concluded, "We need further study looking at real people to see if the blood-brain barrier is affected. If this happens it could lead to disturbances, such as headaches, feeling tired, or problems with sleeping, maybe even things much more serious down the line."

The study drew attention around the world. Colin Roy, the director of the nonionizing-radiation branch of the Australian Radiation Protection and Nuclear Safety Agency, noted: "If radio frequency radiation, or radiation like that of mobile phones, has effects on the blood-brain barrier, then certainly for human health that is quite important."

In response to Leszczynski's 2002 work, Jo-Anne Basile of the Cellular Telecommunications Industry Association repeated the position that industry has taken for the past four decades — we need more research. Who could argue?

I asked Leszczynski about this study during his visit to Washington, D.C., when he testified before the U.S. Senate in September 2010. He recalled, "The reason this finding was so upsetting was not that we proved that cell phones were bad for you, but that we clearly showed that radiation from a phone had a biological impact. After this work, which in fact repeated that of many others and was done in our laboratories, the world could no longer pretend that the only problems with cell phones occurred after you could measure a change in temperature. This view was always mistaken, of course, and our work showed that."

The "hot hypothesis" remains the linchpin of all regulatory guidelines regarding cell phones around the world today. A major disconnect exists. Most people are completely unaware that radio frequency radiation causes any biological impact. I believe self-censorship has created a disconnect within the scientific community as well.

A Driver Of Economic Growth

Leszczynski has been invited to work in China because Chinese officials understand the powerful ways that radio frequency radiation is transforming their own economy and that they need to find out what impacts it may be having on their health as well. I first visited Shanghai in the mid 1980s. In the past decade Shanghai and Beijing have had more than half of the world's construction cranes working to erect as many high-rise buildings as they could. If you close your eyes and open them in downtown Shanghai, you see a skyline that for a moment appears to be that of any large metropolitan city in the Western world. You see buildings emblazoned with names like Motorola, Hewlett-Packard, Cisco Systems, and Google — although that company's presence is in retreat, at least for now. China is the world's largest market of cell phone users — more than one billion.

A similar growth is evident in India. Bangalore has become a growth phenomenon akin to Silicon Valley a decade or so ago. Phones in Bangalore have been banned in schools for years. It is illegal to sell a phone to someone under the age of sixteen, but the law is often ignored. So much so that in April 2010, the city issued new rules restricting cell phone use in schools by students — and teachers. The reasons for these limits on phones are both physical and social. There are mounting concerns that phones can undermine the educational environment. All over the world today, students may sit with their hands in their laps, holding phones that they don't need to look at and sending text messages rather than paying attention to whatever is going on around them. Texting sends out less radiation than talking, but it still isn't a good idea to hold a cell phone in your lap.

The powerful economic and social benefits of cell phone technology are obvious in China and around the developing world, from remote Kenyan villages in Africa to fishing communities in Asia. University of California, Los Angeles, Professor Robert Jensen has shown how cell phones dramatically improved the efficiency of the local fishing industry. The European Union reports that cell phones are major drivers of development across many sectors in both developed and developing nations.

In those times before cell phones had become a global market, as long as five years ago, development economists used to say that if you taught a man to fish, you've fed him for life. Of course, entrepreneurial success as a fisherman depends on there being a steady supply of, say, fish and the means to process and sell them. Today cell phones are making all kinds of commercial enterprises more efficient, enabling the delivery of goods and services. A new proverb for the age might be "Give a village woman a cell phone, and you have seeded local and regional economic booms." Farmers are using phones to decide when to plant crops, what supplies they need, what bank to use to borrow or lend money, and where they get the best prices for their products.

Young criminals in Nairobi employ cell phones to send prostitutes and drugs where limited police presence cannot be found. And the use of cell phones has dramatically changed the ability of law enforcement to track and capture unsophisticated thieves and black marketers who don't yet realize how easy it is to follow their whereabouts by zinging directly into the location of their phones.

It all adds up to bigger gross domestic product numbers.

An Inspired Insider

Stephen C. is the sort of man you would love to have as your next door neighbor. Because he was a math and science whiz as an undergraduate, he was tapped to become a network engineer and rose to great corporate heights working for a company he cannot name. The company supported his obtaining his MBA from Harvard and promoted him to director of one of its most sensitive projects. At one point he had his own big city apartment and lavish allowances for business expenses, and the wardrobe and wine cellar that go with that. Married for thirty-two years to his high school sweetheart, he plays the piano, loves photography, and is now embarking on a new career in parks and recreation. After years of international travel and developing some unsettling health problems of his own, he burned out.

Trained as a network engineer in 1977, Stephen started out working for the banking industry, designing the wires and cables needed to go to different banks and branches and trading terminals. All these networks were hardwired. "I would be called in to design the system. We'd need to understand what machines they were using, what sorts of circuits they had already, their planned growth and future needs.

"We tried to push the first video phones. Nothing really happened. I don't know if people were just not ready for it. The phones were big and bulky and people really didn't think that they needed to see somebody to talk to them. It was way ahead of its time and it was very expensive for the units, and you couldn't have just one. You needed to have two to see something. That's when I understood that the market has to be ubiquitous in order for it to be accepted."

By the 1990s, the world was ready for wireless.

"At that time, I was starting to get into international work and there was a huge demand because the infrastructure was so poor in developing countries. From a military perspective, there was an interest in connecting isolated bases, everything from the White House on down wanted secure wireless — that was the big thing, especially for the military and executive branches of the government. The key with wireless, it wasn't so much that you were untethered as some of the applications — they changed lives. These were exciting times for all of us. I loved the international work I did, such as setting up antennas in places that did not have running water.

"I remember the sheer joy on the face of this one woman in South Africa's KwaZulu-Natal province. When she saw that she could talk to her sister, whom she had not seen in six years, by using this phone, she laughed and cried. Straightaway she got down to business and they had set up a way to find out how many purses made out of discarded plastic could be sold in Cape Town. When I came back a year later, that woman had a television set and indoor plumbing. This was microcredit and technology in action. The small loan she got to pay for that phone became a source of real growth for her and her family."

According to the Geneva-based International Telecommunication Union, the number of cell phones in Africa rose almost ten-fold in the first five years of the twenty-first century, from 15.6 to 135 million. In addition to economic growth in poor villages, there is yet another benefit of cell phones to African women, who have traditionally been the least advantaged on the continent. In this same province, rural women are using cell phones to report violations of their human rights. The UmNyango Project literally means "doorway" in Zulu-Natal, and was established by Fahamu, a pan-African organization based in Cape Town, Nairobi, Dakar, and Oxford.

Making Big Cities Back Home Safer Too?

Stephen returned from his successes in Africa to a promotion. He was brought in to lead a team of a hundred people who would see that the large American city where he worked would never go through the communications nightmare of New York City in the aftermath of the 9/11 terrorist attack. Police and fire departments were literally unable to communicate with one another because they did not share the same wavelength.

The solution to this problem was simple — find a wavelength that could be used exclusively for public safety and make sure to build enough antennas for everyone to get on as if there were an emergency all the time. This was an exciting and important project and he was proud to be involved. But then he became concerned. "At that point some of the public schools we had approached to build antennas on began to balk. Citizens were concerned about what all that higher power radiation might mean for their kids. I thought these were reasonable concerns and I said we needed to look into this. After all, we are operating in a dense city and maybe there was a way to reduce exposures. That's when my job started to get difficult.

"Without saying I was on my way out, they brought in a guy to replace me, who was supposed to basically conduct a public relations effort. He did. He turned to a religious institution, which was glad to accept payment for putting antennas on their schools without ever consulting their communities."

After a while, he began to develop strange problems. "I used to drive my car and have my phone right next to my ear and my ear would get warm. I thought about it: I have these one-sided symptoms, like pain behind my eye and migraines, maybe it's my age — I was just forty then. They were always on the same side that I held my phone. It would hurt behind my eye. I went to the doctor and they did MRIs and didn't find anything.

"At that time, my children were teenagers when they first got their phones. I told them to be careful about having them close to their head all the time. I didn't know what it might be, but I figured it made sense from what I felt was going on and made sure that they used earpieces even when nobody else did.

"I began to ask questions at headquarters that people didn't like my asking. I wondered, if you are not supposed to be around an antenna when it's on, how can it be safe to have a small base station or a booster system for wireless in your own home?

"I had been thrilled to promote a technology that I know saves lives and helps lift people out of poverty. But I grew very uneasy, as I was being asked to help promote the spread of technology into places where nobody could tell us whether it's really safe. It's one thing to put up antennas in remote areas of the African savannah and another to install thousands of them in a single square mile of a major city. I also asked whether we should reduce the power of antennas being put on stoplights that send the radiation directly down onto the street and the people below."

The African Story Nobody Likes To Tell

Few people ever think about what goes into building a cell phone. But it turns out that one component is a relatively rare and expensive mineral called coltan, short for columbite-tantalite, a metallic ore comprising niobium and tantalum, found mainly in the eastern regions of the Democratic Republic of Congo (formerly Zaire). When refined, coltan resists heat and can store an electrical charge — two very important properties for today's phones or for circuit boards inside computers.

Under conditions unchanged for three hundred years, in Congo today coltan is mined as gold and diamonds were, by groups of boys and men digging by hand in streams, scraping off the surface mud. Coltan ore settles at the bottom of a small pond, where about one kilo a day can be extracted.

As part of the technology boom in the late 1990s, the price of coltan skyrocketed ten-fold to $600 U.S. per kilogram. The rush to find coltan also fueled child labor and environmental havoc. In order to mine the mineral, huge swaths of pristine riverbeds were cleared of all vegetation and animal life. Among the carnage was our primate cousin — those prized gorillas of the mist that Dian Fossey had made so famous. The coltan mining zone includes Kahuzi-Biega National Park, home of the mountain gorilla, whose population has been halved by the mining operation. The UN Environment Programme reports that the number of eastern lowland gorillas in all national parks of Congo has dropped 90 percent over the past five years, and only three thousand now survive.

While the world has tolerated various forms of servitude of poor African boys and girls for centuries as being culturally inevitable, it no longer accepts the killing of gorillas. As a result an international campaign was launched. In fact, the rewards of coltan mining are considerable, as a typical miner can earn twenty times more than the usual Congolese worker's salary of ten U.S. dollars per month. In response to public uproar over the devastating impact of coltan mining on gorillas, the American-based Kemet, the world's largest maker of tantalum capacitors, asked its suppliers to certify that their coltan ore does not come from the Democratic Republic of Congo or from neighboring countries. Whether this will lead to "gorilla safe" cell phones being marketed, much like "dolphin safe" tuna, remains to be seen.

For the past decade, civil wars over the rich minerals of the region have wracked the country, killing more than three million. Mvemba Phezo Dizolele reported for the Pulitzer Crisis Center from the Mishangu Hills, where children as young as seven work with archaic mortars and pestles, chipping the mineral away from eighty-million-year-old hard rock in open pits and belowground mines. A substantial amount of the world's supply of this mineral comes from a region where rape is a common war tactic and internecine struggles have gone on for decades. This mineral has become the new blood diamond in the Great Lakes areas of Africa. A recent report by the

UN has claimed that all the parties involved in the local civil war have been involved in the mining and sale of coltan. One report suggested that the neighboring Rwandan army made

U.S. $250 million in less than eighteen months from selling coltan, despite there being no coltan in Rwanda to mine. The military forces of Uganda and Burundi are also implicated in smuggling coltan out of Congo for resale in Belgium.

New Business

On one of the last mornings I was finishing up the writing of this book, three young men phoned me on a conference call, excited about what they had invented. Indeed, they have patented a product that sounds fascinating. They are not brain scientists but businessmen. One has a fresh doctorate in applied mathematics and another is an attorney. One is the first person in his family to go to college. They hail from my hometown region in the Monongahela Valley of western Pennsylvania. I imagine some very proud parents.

"When I was doing my doctoral research at MIT, I figured out there has got to be a way to reduce the amount of radiation going into the brain and out of the phone, by using some secret materials that I can't tell you about," Jeff, the mathematician, informed me Jeff played football for a major Ivy League school on a full scholarship and actually was drafted by the NFL, getting out before he got badly hurt. He had developed headaches that wouldn't go away until he started using an earpiece. Could be a coincidence, but he doesn't think so. So he began talking to the others about how to make a better, safer phone.

"We figure that it can't be good for you to hold a microwave radio next to your brain. We know that cell phones are revolutionary, and that they are here to stay. We are going to make them safer. Our invention will reduce radiation into the head, and increase the amount going out more safely."

Others are already working on redesigning phones so that their antennas use less power, or that rely on a different wavelength altogether. After all, there are much shorter wavelengths that do not vibrate with the human body or make people hear sounds inside their heads. I have no idea whether any of these devices work, but I believe these young men, or businesspeople like them, have the creativity to accomplish this goal. And I believe markets around the world will reward them.

Despite our growing dependency on phones for many functions of our daily lives, it makes no sense to continue assuming that today's phones are safe based on standards that were created for large men who didn't use them very much and when current technologies did not exist. One thing is clear at this point: Cell phones have become as essential to modern life as cars and trucks and jet planes. We spend billions of dollars, euros, yen, and yuan making vehicles safer for us to drive or fly in and checking to see if they are safe as used. We need to do the same things with cell phones. Rather than parroting assurances of safety based on old science, outmoded theories of physics, and bullied scientists, we need to invest in cell phones' safety as we do with other modern technologies.

Of course, more research is needed. On that we are all agreed. But the need for research should not be allowed to become an excuse to carry on as though everything is fine, until we have incontrovertible proof that it is not. Yes, we do not have an epidemic of brain tumors in countries that have used cell phones heavily for little more than a decade. But ten years after cigarettes began to be heavily smoked, we also did not have an epidemic of lung cancer.

Years from now our grandchildren will look back and ask: Did we do the right thing and act to protect them, or did we harm them needlessly, irresponsibly, and permanently, blinded by the addictive delights of our technological age?

12

WHAT NOW? (2010)

The genie is out of the bottle and is not going back.

When the hardcover edition of this book went to press in the summer of 2010, the issue of cell phones and health fell under the public radar and outside the scientific mainstream. As this paperback goes to press, the era when cell phone safety was taken for granted is over. The science confirming that pulsed digital microwave radiation from cell phones changes biology and can be harmful has become stronger and clearer. Cell phone science and safety questions have garnered global attention from the British and Israeli governments, major television and radio networks, and from a wide range of publications including *the Journal of the American Medical Association, Time, the Wall Street Journal, the Guardian, the Economist, Haaretz, China Daily, the Indian Times, the Globe and Mail* (in both Britain and Canada), *Scientific American*, and *Green American*. Sales of headsets and landlines and the practice of texting are up while sales of phones to young children are dropping in many quarters. At the time of writing, a newly revised pamphlet released by the U.K. Health Department advises all to text rather than talk and affirms previous advice that children under age sixteen limit their use of phones.

Still, the fight to frame the discussion continues. The term manufacturers give to cell phone emissions — radio frequency energy — suggests a benign and harmless by-product. After all, radios are pleasant music-playing devices and energy is something we all want to have. An alternative phrase is both the truth and more useful: microwave radiation. Microwaves encompass wavelengths that can cook food because they heat up fluids, and include the frequencies operating every single one of the world's five billion cell phones: between 800 MHz and 2,400 MHz (the latter being the frequency used to power baby monitors, garage-door openers, wireless routers, cordless and cell phones, though only cell phones and cordless phones are typically held close to the brain and body).

The cell phone industry has argued against using the word radiation to describe their chief products. In San Francisco, where legislators tried implementing the Cell Phone Radiation Disclosure Law, also known as the Right-to-Know ordinance, the Cellular Telecommunications Industry Association (CTIA) insisted that people will become confused by referring to cell phones as two-way microwave radiating devices. In their suit to block this new law, the CTIA claimed that all phones are equally safe.

While the FCC once advised those concerned about reducing exposures to purchase lower SAR phones, on the eve of public hearings on the matter in the city of Burlingame, California, the government Web site underwent an about-face. With no advance request for comment or public notice, the FCC questioned the value of any reliance on the SAR. Even if SAR for one phone is low and higher for another, the CTIA and FCC now agree, this provides no value to the consumer.

Their safety depends on how you use them. Phones used in areas with poor signal strength will release more radiation, so therefore SAR alone is useless. In truth, even for the *same* phone, the amount of radiation released depends on which carrier frequency it uses.

As a measure of maximum radiation absorbed, SAR remains a flawed, even crude concept, but one that provides a useful metric nonetheless. In truth, the SAR makes little difference if the cell phone or cordless phone is kept even a slight distance away from the head and body. If a person uses a phone with a high SAR value, she is more likely than not to be exposed to more radiation than if she uses a phone with a low SAR value. SAR is just like information we get from fuel efficiency ratings for new cars. We all know that actual mileage varies quite a bit from what is posted on the vehicles in the showroom. But it is still useful to know that one car has an average reported 40 MPG rating, while another has half that. Why should we be denied the same information about potential microwave radiation from cell phones?

Recent widely publicized reports from psychiatrist Nora Volkow, the acclaimed chief of the National Institute of Drug Abuse, have fundamentally changed the nature of public discourse. Her work reveals that contrary to U.S. government assumptions that cell phone radiation produces no biological impact on the living brain, just fifty minutes of exposure to a cell phone held next to the head of a healthy adult significantly alters the amount of glucose — the brain's main fuel. Whether or not these brain changes prove to be temporary or permanent and what their repeated occurrence portends are matters that cannot be ignored.

Too much glucose in the brain or bloodstream provides a nutritional matrix that encourages the growth of bacteria or viruses, which can make wound healing quite difficult in those with diabetes, and may also underlie the brains of those with Alzheimer's. An excess of glucose could also lead to a kind of burnout in the engines of sperm (mitochondria) and may goad the growth of cancerous cells.

The Volkow study is not the world-changing scientific development the news media has portrayed. In 1994 Henry Lai and N. P. Singh showed that pulsed microwave radiation to the brains of rats mutate brain DNA. It was the first demonstration of what has since become an important tool in basic research that is now applied to many compounds — the comet assay, a technique that images the unraveling of DNA. At the time of their studies, these two University of Washington researchers were not aware of earlier work from the 1970s showing that microwave signals weakened the blood-brain barrier, nor did they appreciate that plans were under way to mass-market cell phones. Their research proved inconvenient to those concerned with creating demand for these new devices. That was why some industry representatives first sought to keep the findings of Lai and Singh from being published and why other industry representatives had gone to the journal editor that had accepted this peer-reviewed paper for publication and requested that it be unaccepted. Others wrote to the National Institutes of Health and the University of Washington alleging that research funds had been misused.

When all these efforts to discredit their work failed, Motorola decided on what it described as a "war-gaming" set of public relations initiatives against the results (according to a memo released by Microwave News that was originally sent by the company's head of global affairs to a firm hired for precisely this purpose).

In fact, Volkow's widely publicized work is part of a long tradition of studies that have found that cell phone radiation — whether from older or newer phones — significantly alters brain chemistry and blood flow. In 2006, Finnish researchers produced similar results of altered brain energy after cell phone use; and in 2002 researchers in Austria presented parallel evidence of other significant changes, briefly capturing the same headlines, "Cell Phone Radiation Affects the Brain," albeit in German.

Fast-forward to 2011. Remember those accusations of fraud made against the REFLEX project — the twelve-laboratory European collaboration headed by Franz Adlkofer — after they found further evidence that cell phone radiation induced biological damage? Exonerated by several internal university reviews, recently that work was further strengthened when yet another investigation found no evidence of fraud. New research from Israel's Weizmann Institute and from Chinese and Japanese investigators can be found on the Environmental Health Trust Web site and has confirmed and extended the REFLEX results: pulsed digital microwave radiation damages DNA and produces other biological changes that often predict cancer. 3-G phones appear worse than 2-G phones, although mechanisms remain unclear.

Science is profoundly more social than most appreciate. In the seventeenth century, the convicted heretic Galileo was forced to recant his notion that the earth moved around the sun and live out his life under house arrest. In the nineteenth century, the breakthrough experiments by the humble, self-taught Michael Faraday showing the ties between magnetism and electricity were dismissed as charlatanism. Today, hypotheses linking pulsed microwave radiation from cell phones to various types of biological damage are moving from the rarefied world of little-known research to the foundation for landmark shifts in public perception and, ultimately, life-saving policies. The assumption that cell phones cannot have a biological impact — unless they produce a measureable change in temperature — which underlies the standards set for the world's five billion phones, is plain wrong.

While cutting-edge science is continuing to evolve, the policy debate has begun to shift. Based on its own review of the matter, in 2010 the President's Cancer Panel (whose members were appointed by President George W. Bush), drawing on what it heard from me and other experts in the field about growing rates of rare tumors that could be tied with cell phones, called for both serious research and precautionary actions on cell phones and other wireless devices. Yet the rest of the government has not received that memo. No monitoring of human impacts of cell phone radiation is planned or under way in North America. Invoking decade-old research, official government Web sites continue to offer assurances of safety, using language that is eerily similar to that employed by the cell phone industry. Nowadays government Web sites also contain information about how you can reduce your exposure to cell phone radiation — but add that there's really no need to do so.

A growing number of the world's leading experts are issuing calls for protective policies. Michael Kundi, head of the Medical University of Vienna's Institute of Environmental Health, speaking on behalf of the BioInitiative Working Group in 2011, concludes that new findings that consistently show lowered sperm count and quality, a doubled risk of brain cancer, and hearing damage after a decade of regular cell phone use, require us to avoid future risks now.

In urging precautionary actions, Kundi and I are not alone.

Two leaders of the World Health Organization Interphone study — the largest research study to date on brain tumor risks from cell phones, which took four years to carry out and ten years to be published — have also broken ranks with those who claim we have no cause for concern. Elisabeth Cardis, Ph.D., of Barcelona's Centre for Research in Environmental Epidemiology, and Siegal Sadetzki, M.D., M.P.H., of Tel Aviv's Gertner Institute for Epidemiology and Health Policy, note the following in a publication of the British Medical Association from early 2011:

> *While more studies are needed to confirm or refute these results, indications of an increased risk [of brain cancer] in high and long-term users from Interphone and other studies are of concern. . . . Even a small risk at the individual level could eventually result in a considerable number of tumors and become an important public-health issue. Simple and low-cost*

*measures, such as the use of text messages, hands-free kits, and/
or the loudspeaker mode of the phone could substantially reduce
exposure to the brain from mobile phones. Therefore, until
definitive scientific answers are available, the adoption of such
precautions, particularly among young people, is advisable.*

They also note that most research on cell phone radiation and
brain tumors has focused on those who used their phones for a few
hours a month for less than five years and no studies had examined
effects on children.

WHO experts are in accord with the cautionary measures suggested in this book and by the Israeli Health and Environment Min-
istries, the French National Assembly, the European Environment
Agency, and many others — including the authors of "Cellphones
and Brain Tumors: 15 Reasons for Concern" (see www.radiationre-
search.org) and recent reports from neurosurgeons Charles Teo and
Vini Khurauna in Australia, Kevin O'Neill in Britain, and Santosh
Kesari and Keith Black in the United States. (Please see "Doctors'
Advice to Patients and Their Families," which is available at www.
ehtrust.org.)

Andrea Boland, the independent legislator from Maine who first
galvanized national U.S. attention, is reintroducing her call for warning labels on cell phones. This is a call that many are now taking up
across our nation and around the world, including Philadelphia's city-
wide councilwoman Blondell Reynolds Brown, Pennsylvania State
representative Vanessa Lowery Brown, and British and Canadian
members of Parliament. Bipartisan support recently has come from
the states of Oregon, Montana, California, and Wyoming, and towns
ranging from Jackson Hole, Wyoming, to Burlingame and Berkeley,
California, and Portland, Maine — all of which are informing their
citizens about the need to take basic precautions. Mayor Mark Baron

quips, "Look, we don't have all the answers. But should the lack of major health problems now keep us from doing what seems sensible and simple to do in protecting ourselves and our kids?"

More than forty years ago, well before cell phones existed, Allan Frey showed that the notion that microwave radiation had to produce heat to create damage was flat-out wrong.

Frey found many different effects of microwave radiation, from weakening the blood-brain barrier to increasing the uptake of drugs against leukemia; from interfering with heartbeats, hearing, or learning to stimulating opioid receptors like those that cause addiction. Volkow's work suggests that altered glucose metabolism may be the common thread underlying the biological effects that Frey demonstrated decades ago. It's an intriguing possibility that will only be resolved if and when a truly independent research program is established.

A simple dollar a phone fee for the next five years — something I called for in testimony before the Senate in 2009 — will allow us to determine any problems with existing phones and the need to improve technology. In the meantime, phones need warning labels saying that they do emit microwave radiation, and people have a right to know the relative SAR number of every phone, just like they can learn sodium content, fuel efficiency, and fat content from reading food labels. But no matter how low the SAR may be on any phone, when a phone is connecting to towers for signals, it should never be held next to the brain or body.

Public perception in some quarters is changing, but the disconnect persists. Federal regulations have not been significantly revised for close to two decades.

Here's what the FCC Web site says about children and cell phones as of April 1, 2011: "The scientific evidence does not show a danger to any users of cell phones from RF exposure, including children and teenagers."

It is time for a change.

13

CAN YOU HEAR ME NOW?

Science is the search for truth that is the effort to understand the world: it involves the rejection of bias, of dogma, of revelation, but not the rejection of morality.

~Linus Pauling

When *Disconnect* was first published more than a decade ago, my seasoned agent, Al Zuckerman, had been guardedly optimistic. Al, whose clients included best-selling novelists Ken Follett and Nora Roberts, as well as Stephen Hawking — the modern-day Einstein — felt we were onto something big. He also had personal reasons to hope we would quickly achieve critical acceptance. He had just begun to compete for real face time with family members so enthralled with their cell phones they would not look him in the eye. My publisher and the senior editor at Penguin Dutton, Stephen Morrow, had a similar agenda — he was deeply concerned about impacts on his then-young toddlers.

We all expected the successes of my previous works boded well for this new one. Previous appearances on PBS, Fox News, Living on Earth, CNN, BBC, and with Dr. Oz, Larry King, Sanjay Gupta, Terry Gross, and Diane Rehm suggested there would be a ready market for this work, as did my associations at many universities in the United States and elsewhere.

We were mistaken. Producers with whom I had worked for decades did not return phone calls. Where the Heinz Family Endowment handed out two thousand copies of my book, *The Secret History of the War on Cancer*, to academic conferences and galas in Boston and Pittsburgh, and where the New York Academy of Sciences had published excerpts from that work, no such sponsorship emerged for *Disconnect.*

How Little I Knew

Writing comes from a conviction that somebody cares enough to take the time to read whatever it is we have taken the time to commit to paper. Noam Chomsky has stated, "The general population doesn't know what's happening, and it doesn't even know that it doesn't know." This statement can certainly be applied to the public's knowledge of wireless radiation dangers. Certainly the first edition of this book came from my own shock at realizing how little I knew about how the brain reacts to erratic microwave radiation-emitting devices often held next to our heads. As someone who had held a senior post at the U.S. National Academy of Sciences and taught at major universities, I assumed that if there were a real problem, my colleagues and I would know about it.

As I began to explore the science, I learned that a number of respected authorities had tried to tackle the issue years earlier and found their hands tied. The prolific award-winning *New York Times* science reporter, B. Blake Levitt, and her brilliant predecessor Paul Brodeur, had documented risks from electromagnetic radiation in a series of articles and books that surely should have been candidates for the Pulitzer Prize. Their work and other indications that such radiation could be harmful never managed to fuel broad public discussions. Instead, as I reported in *Disconnect*, any report on potential harm from cell phones is treated just like the early study completed by University of Washington Professor Henry Lai and Narenda Singh in 1994 (done long before cell phones were in broad use). That study, which showed that wireless radiation can damage brain cells, became a topic to be "war-gamed," as the never-repudiated 1994 memo from Motorola to their public relations agency advised.

In 2007, the *BioInitiative Report* provided a major comprehensive review by some of the world's top scientists in the field of bioelectromagnetics. That report continues to be regularly updated online with the latest relevant science, as does our website ehtrust. org. Industry confidants advise that well over $250,000 per year had then been allocated at the time to efforts to dismiss the science of this report, along with the science behind the World Health Organization's 2011 declaration that cell phone radiation constitutes a possible human carcinogen. These serious reports detailing the public health risks of wireless radiation were regarded as nothing more than highly inconvenient public relations problems. War-gaming the science has been going on for decades, carefully manufacturing doubts about the science.

My Own Lifestyle Changes

In 2005, I was Director of the Center for Environmental Oncology at the University of Pittsburgh Cancer Institute. I had started out wearing two BlackBerry phones at my hips — kind of like a gunslinger — as did many of my scientific colleagues. We were proud to be so important that we needed to be always on call and able to interrupt one another's private lives with whatever idea popped into our heads at any moment. Within a few months of looking into the matter, those two cell phones were relegated to my desk or my purse and never again held against my body.

While we cannot simply combine information on the growing

number of cell phone user survivors and non-survivors to prove the science about cell phone radiation hazards, their personal stories reveal compelling details about the range of impacts phones can wield in modern life. For all these individual tales of death and illness, the unifying theme is very simple — frequent and heavy use of cell phones or other wireless radiating devices was their habit before the onset of their maladies. Each single instance of illness is, of course, unique. Nevertheless, such examples form part of a larger whole portrayed in this book.

I must begin, of course, with my Pittsburgh colleague the best-selling author and neuropsychiatrist David Servan-Schreiber, who was dead of brain cancer just one year after he penned the first foreword to this book in 2010. Until we had met as leaders of our respective programs at the University of Pittsburgh medical systems, when he was 47, David Servan-Schreiber had been a proud self-pro-nounced cell phone addict, starting a new life with a young wife and family. Like many hard-charging, highly productive people, he had loved the capacity to be always on. Beginning with the earliest and highest-powered and radiating phones, from morning to night, the moment the wheels hit the tarmac at the airport, in trains, elevators, taxis, or buses, David had been easily accessible, engaging, and chat-tering away on one of his three phones.

Years before at the tender age of 31, when his grad student unex-pectedly did not show up for a test run, David hopped into the latest brain research tool of Carnegie Mellon — the magnetic resonance imaging machine. That might have saved his life at that time as it allowed his colleagues to discover a tiny white patch of brain cancer that was quickly removed. Combining the best conventional and unconventional medicine, David kept that cancer at bay for 18 years. This was noteworthy in itself and became the basis for his best-selling book, *Anticancer*, published in more than a dozen languages and still available in a new edition today.

In 2011, that streak ended. He had phoned me early one morning from Paris, right after he got the news. He sounded breathless.

"I wanted to let you know. The MRI shows I've got a big tumor in the brain. Of course, I'm fine." He paused.

"I'm fine. Really. Now," he repeated as though the words would make it all true. "I rode my bike home through the streets right after I got the results."

"What? It must be 11 p.m. Did you ride your bike at night through Paris? Did you have a helmet?" I stammered.

He laughed. "No, of course not. At this point, I figured I had bigger risks to worry about than crashing my bike."

Just one month after that phone call, we sat together in the sunny 18th century drawing room of his home. David's partner Gwen floated in. With her big, beautiful seven-month pregnant belly and a Mona Lisa smile, she seemed like an actor entering the wrong set. Their toddler son's toys filled the area where we drank tea.

"Now," David sighed. "Now, they will say that all my ideas about preventing cancer are worthless. That I failed."

"But, David," I rejoined, "there are so many things that affect the chance of brain cancer. There's no way to know whether this cancer has anything to do with the old one. Perhaps this is a new cancer altogether."

"Yes," he admitted.

"Have you thought about all those cell phone calls, all that microwave radiation that entered your head at peak power over many years around the world? You know that holding a phone smack against your head as you travel uses your head as a microwave antenna?

"We don't know how to reverse the damage those calls may have made. All the green tea, fish, walnuts, avocado, and blueberries in the world might not be enough. Remember, as you move in a car with the phone held at your head the signal always goes to maximum power as it connects to each next tower along the way so the signal is not lost," I blurted out.

David replied. "We can never know. Yes, we can never know. But *you, you* had better find out!"

Since the first edition of this book in 2010, the mounting losses of people like David, at a mere fifty years of age, feel especially senseless. Yes, for eighteen years David had survived one form of brain cancer. As to the precise role that cell phone radiation played in producing or promoting his fatal glioblastoma multiforme brain cancer, we know a lot more now than we did when he was first diagnosed.

Alan and Ellie Marks. The launch of *Disconnect* at the Commonwealth Club in 2010, was an astonishing event. I will never forget those who came to the standing room-only event in the blue-velvet curtained main conference room that day. Passionate, fiery, and articulate, Ellie Marks had helped organize the event. She was angry then and is angrier now. Her husband Alan's first seven-hour-long surgery in 2008 removed a mass from the right side of his brain where he usually held his phone. That same year, she testified before Congressman Dennis Kucinich regarding the compelling connection of cell phone use with her husband's brain cancer. As a top California realtor, Alan used mobile phones for more than ten hours daily, starting in the 1990s. With a charismatic personality that no one can say "no" to, Ellie became an invaluable resource for me and many others. With Ellie's leadership, the Commonwealth Club event in 2010 provided a chance to convene several other brave people who wanted to use the book launch to tell the world their heartbreaking stories. If nothing else took place that entire year, seeing the haunting faces of those who had lost their sons and daughters, fathers and mothers gave me a determination that will not and cannot quit.

Ellie became EHT's Director of Government Relations and earned battle scars opposing the telecom industry over California's Right to

Know laws. She would go on to found the California Brain Tumor Association. CABTA, along with a growing number of other groups, has played a lead role in promoting public awareness of increased concerns through its relentless efforts to advance a legislative agenda (posted on EHT's website). Fortunately, Ellie has become even more determined and focused on seeing the world learn from and be spared her family's struggles with Alan's brain cancer.

Alan is one of the longest-standing survivors of this horrible disease, having endured multiple surgeries and other interventions. While Ellie did much public talk on the subject, Alan has said, "I wish I had known I was killing myself by using my phone."

Brett Bocook. When we first met at San Francisco's Commonwealth Club in 2010, Brett looked like a movie star. Six foot five and about 195 pounds with dark curly black hair and a smile that lit up the room, Brett appeared pretty much like the magnetic, fit national rowing champion he had once been. Like one of Central Casting's calls for a bright, attractive, powerful attorney, he was the perfect California boy. A varsity crew leader, he had trained for the Olympics hours a day, building strength with a metal harness tied to a huge hook that allowed him to haul a truck around the block.

A few months before our Commonwealth Club event, his world crashed when he collapsed in the shower from a seizure. As a practicing attorney, he calculated he had used his cell phone for one million minutes in his lifetime. One million minutes. A non-smoker, he was the textbook case of someone who had lived a good healthy life yet ended up with a terrible disease. His heart stopped beating twice when he collapsed in the shower. His dazzling smile and head of hair that many women adore and many men envy stood in stark contrast to the shaved half of his skull, finely etched with a neatly stapled semi-circular incision carved to excise a brain tumor.

An expert in patent law, Bocook discovered that the industry had filed numerous patents to reduce electromagnetic radiation dating from the 1990s.

"They know. They know," he said. "They have known for years that they need to reduce that radiation. That's why they have all these patents on making technology safer. But they will not apply for them until and unless they are legally forced to do so."

Bocook walked out of a study on brain cancer that he had agreed to be enrolled in after that researcher put him through a two-hour interview and did not ask a single question about cell phone use. He was outraged but not surprised.

"Who do you think funds this research? It's safer to blame everything on chemicals like they did with Gulf War cases, including Beau Biden. But everybody knows it is not chemicals or cell phones, and it will turn out to be both. Follow the money and you will see that the telecom industry is the most generous funder on both sides of the political aisle and one of the biggest advertisers in all media. So no wonder it's so hard to get the story out!" he declared.

"But nobody's gonna stop me!"

In 2015, right after his fifth surgery he was back in training. This time using a walker.

"They got it out, while I was awake," he beamed proudly when we visited the University of San Francisco Medical Center Hospital in November.

"Let's go for a spin. I've got wheels," he piped as he strode next to me, gripping his upright metal stroller that held his intravenous pole.

Convinced he would be in the small number of patients that survive brain cancer for a decade, he fathered a baby born in 2015 — the same year he died. Brett's brief but spectacular story can be found along with others on Environmental Health Trust's website under "cell phone survivors and non-survivors."

Jimmy Gonzalez. Attorney Jimmy Gonzalez was a comet who crossed my path determined to tell the world — in Spanish and English radio broadcasts we did together — that long-term constant cell phone use had given him brain cancer in 2011. Charming, articulate, and very handsome, this former U.S. Marine Corps officer and attorney stared down brain cancer that occurred where he had held his phone. The father of young children and husband of an attorney, Gonzalez was determined to take a right to know to his community in 2012, angered by the rank power plays with which industry had upended California efforts.

"If I had ever been told the truth — that a cell phone is a two-way microwave radio," he once quipped, "I would have been crazy to have kept it next to my brain."

Like David Servan-Schreiber, when Gonzalez talked, people listened. He could not be dismissed as fringy or uninformed. He was tough. He had survived Marine Corps basic training of the "Crucible" — a four-day-long, sleep-deprived, physically challenging test of stamina, courage, and psychological grit training program that was canceled due to deaths and severe injuries. Like my own son, Aaron, Gonzalez made it through with flying colors. He knew the meaning of the Marine Corps slogan: *the few, the proud.* A George Washington University Law School graduate, Gonzalez practiced in northern Florida.

Gonzalez had applied his legal skills to drafting what would become the Town Council of Jackson, Wyoming, Cell Phone Safety Declaration. Lacking any mandatory components, it handily passed unanimously in 2011. With his earnest, intelligent, and honest pleas, among those paying close attention to Gonzalez's story was the entire governing body of his hometown of Pembroke Pines, Florida. Shortly after hearing Gonzalez's presentation of his troubling story, the Pembroke Pines council members passed their proclamation informing their citizens of the right to know how to use cell phones safely. He died on November 27, 2014, leaving a widow, young children, and a YouTube video of his poignant testimony.

Tiffany Frantz. I met Tiffany and her mom Traci in 2012 shortly after the twenty-one year old was diagnosed with cancer that began as tumors directly under the cell phone antennas that she stored in her bra as a young teen. The tumors advanced into her liver, brain, and bones. With no family history and no genetic risk factors for the disease, doctors were convinced that keeping her cell phone next to her skin had caused this highly unusual disease. Traci and Tiffany shared their travails with millions on television appearances, some of which can still be found on YouTube. Despite multiple surgeries, Tiffany managed to find joy in her marriage during which she continued to undergo repeated operations and treatments. Her story, along with scientific studies corroborating the risk to the breast from microwave radiating antennas, forms the foundation for multi-media interactive educational materials developed with the Massachusetts Breast Cancer Coalition aimed at informing young women to not keep phones on the body.

In the midst of this tough struggle Traci wrote an open letter chronicling Tiffany's struggles and strongly endorsing the public right to know laws then pending at the City of San Francisco and later endorsed by the City of Berkeley, California. Her letter ended with this haunting prophetic message:

"The wording that is being advocated for is already in the owner's manual which no one takes the time to read. Cell phone manufacturers KNOW there is a danger otherwise they would not include it in their verbiage. We are only asking for it to be better seen by the consumer at the point of sale for the sole purpose of heeding caution and for nothing more. Have you and your family taken the time to read your owner's manual? Have you and your family heeded the advice your cell phone manufacturer recommends?

"I WISH there would have been a warning on the outside of the box for ALL of us to read. My daughter may not have to fight for her life if it were!!!"

Our colleague, surgeon John West, reported in one publication on four confirmed cases and urged that the bra be declared a no-phone zone. Within two years, we had the names of more than thirty other cases with similar stories — some of which can be seen in videos on EHT's website. Additional scientific proof of human harm has now been provided by a study comparing the phone habits of women with breast cancer to those who do not develop the disease. Taiwanese researchers found that women who carried their cell phone near their chest or waist/abdomen area had fivefold and fourfold risks of breast cancer, respectively, compared to those who stored their phones below their waists. Despite the mounting concerns of medical experts, athletic clothing manufacturers make clothing with pockets for phones without warning that phones are tested at a distance off the body and brain and come with seldom seen notices. Tiffany died in 2021 at age 31.

Cally Pivano. Cally brought sunlight into every room and phone call. In 2016, this charismatic marathoner, youthful grandmother, and much-beloved center of her family's life developed a strange pain in her thigh muscle that doctors found puzzling. Intense physical therapy was not able to help. A scan revealed what none had expected — a rare tumor had wrapped itself around her quadricep — the main muscle of the thigh. Cally asked immediately whether this could have anything to do with the many, many hours she had spent curled up with her laptop pressed to her leg, often heating up the tissue. Unconvinced by those who doubted the association, she began a one-woman campaign to reach out to others, including those of us at EHT, to help people understand that no one should keep such devices directly on their bodies for hours a day.

She wrote in *Medium:*

"I had learned that my cancer may have been caused by radiation yet I had no idea how that applied to me and then it hit me, my laptop. I spent hours upon hours with my laptop on the same thigh where the tumor formed not knowing that it shouldn't touch my body.

"How many of you have read the disclaimer about any of your mobile devices? I never did but when I looked up the disclaimer for my laptop I learned that it should be kept 8 inches away from my body. It's a LAPTOP! Who knew?? The disclaimer for my cell phone says to reduce RF exposure, use hands free options such as speakerphone, text messaging or using the supplied headphones."

Callie developed four different cancers over the years, including the one that claimed her life finally — an inoperable tumor around her heart. Her LinkedIn profile used the moniker "cancer warrior girl." Her blog on her fight can no longer be found. She died at age 57.

Paul Doyon. The Internet makes it possible to meet people from far-off lands and gain some measure of their intelligence. For more than a decade, I've been following the odyssey of Paul Doyon — an American fluent in Japanese who lived in Japan for approximately 20 years. Given the high level of knowledge conveyed in his online writings, I assumed he must have had a doctorate in medicine or cellular biology. That was not the case. His knowledge has been acquired the hard way — as a matter of self-defense. He has an exceptional command of the science evolving in the field of bioelectromagnetics because that is how he has saved his own life. Here's his story:

"Back in 2005, I was extremely sick for six months before I was even aware — let alone even imagined — that the two cell towers within 100 meters of my apartment and the WiFi from my neighbors' apartments bleeding into mine might have

had something to do with the host of symptoms — insomnia, anxiety attacks, loss of appetite, rapid weight loss, excessive thirst, swollen lymph nodes, intestinal disturbances, increased sensitivities, weakened immune system, etc. — I was experiencing at the time. I was living in Fukuoka, Japan, at the time with my wife and son (also experiencing health complaints, though not as severe as mine). I had been experiencing the symptoms of a disease state known as 'Chronic Fatigue Syndrome' (CFS) but was later to learn that the same symptoms described a disease identified by the Russians in the early '70s as 'Microwave Sickness.'

"When we started to realize that wireless exposures were bombarding us and that this might be behind our decline in health, we quickly started searching for and found a log house in a white zone — an area devoid of wireless signals — in the mountains of Saga Prefecture, (about 30 minutes outside of Fukuoka), to move into in order get away from these seemingly health-damaging signals and try to recover our health. My wife (who is Japanese) wrote to all the Japanese media outlets to get some coverage for our newly discovered problem that those seemingly innocuous waves of wireless radiation damaged our health. She received zero replies; they did not want to touch our story.

"When something is out of sight, it is also out of mind — and microwaves from cell phones, cell phone towers, and other wireless-radiation-emitting devices are invisible, tasteless, odorless, and cannot be sensed with touch. Naturally, it is difficult for many — even doctors — to fathom them as being a culprit. Increasingly, people worldwide are starting to wake up to the fact of what is indeed the cause of their previously mysterious symptoms. An increasing number of these people

become noticeably ill when exposed to this invisible source of pollution. Also, people with excessive metal toxicity seem to be particularly sensitive. Progress can be made when people realize the problem and come together to find solutions.

"After moving into the log house, I immediately started to feel better with the disappearance of many symptoms in the first 24-hour period and with most of the rest of my symptoms gradually disappearing over a two-four month period. However, at the time, whenever I would get into cell phone range, these symptoms would start to come back. I would feel intense pressure in my head, and I would feel nauseous. I would feel pain in the lymph nodes under my right arm, my right testicle, and my groin area.

"Fortunately, I found an excellent integrative medical doctor, Dr. Toshihiko Yayama, nearby, and through multiple treatment modalities, I recovered much of my health and became much better able to "tolerate" the EMFs. Unfortunately, the levels of EMFs we are exposed to in our environment has been increasing drastically. I now find that I must live in a very rural area to maintain my health."

Justis James Greto. Thankfully, cancer remains relatively rare in children. Few causes of childhood cancer have been identified, with the notable exceptions of ionizing radiation and some industrial chemicals. Unfortunately, cancers in children, including thyroid, breast, and brain cancers, are on the rise for reasons that generally remain unknown. But they are not unknowable. As this edition was being drafted, I heard from the parents of Justis. Their son had been a typical soccer-playing video-gamer. His bedroom featured a microwave radiating Wi-Fi booster on his nightstand to increase the signal strength from the router downstairs. The booster allowed him to play on his Xbox while ostensibly doing homework on his laptop and talking for hours with his friends on his cell phone. Justis played his Xbox using a wireless headset and controller. When he was done playing, he would use his iPad for another hour or two before bed.

Just four months after being diagnosed, Justis lost his fight against a very rare glioblastoma of the brain. The family dog Leia had died of the same disease six months earlier. His parents realize now that they did not understand the impacts of wireless radiation, which permeated Justis' room, where their dog had also slept. Since his death, they created the website JustisForAll.org not only to honor his memory but also to raise the question in the minds of other parents about the impact of wireless radiation and the need to reduce exposures whenever possible.

His parents Mike and Christen shared their story:

"Justis' tumor was classified as a Grade IV Glioblastoma Multiforme (GBM) — the most aggressive and life-threatening form of brain cancer — this is a terminal diagnosis as Glioblastoma does not typically respond to traditional cancer therapies. ...

"We held onto hope and Justis fought with everything he had but on May 11, 2017, less than four months after being diagnosed, Justis left this earthly world to live in light, eternally. ..."

"Leia and Justis were very close and she spent most of her time with Justis in his room while he played video games and wirelessly streamed his favorite shows. There was a lot of wireless radiation, in Justis' room. ... We are positive that our son and our dog lost their lives due to our lack of understanding. There is no wireless in our home now. Everything is wired."

"Justis taught us so many things throughout his short life. And before he left us he taught us one last thing. He taught us that it's our 'human' connection to each other that makes this world a special place. More often than not, we must put

our phones away and enjoy our time with each other. These 'human' connections supersede any connection that technology can provide."

Those mentioned in these stories are just a fraction of the people who have been brought to the attention of Environmental Health Trust because of the prices that they have paid with their bodies for their use of cell phones and other wireless radiating devices. We do not have statistical evidence in many instances but we have powerful proof when one looks at these cases that what they share are unusual uses and exposures to wireless radiation.

Does this prove that was the cause of their demise?

Proof in science is a well-established concept typically requiring evidence that achieves a statistical significance that there is a less than five percent chance that the finding is not true. This is otherwise known as a level of significance of .05. I present these human faces of the toll of microwave radiation not because they have achieved statistical significance. To the contrary, we often, but not always, lack that level of proof. But we now know enough from toxicology studies to say that when animals are exposed to the same kinds of radiation, they do develop the same rare, highly malignant tumors that are killing more and more people today. Do we wait like we did with tobacco and asbestos?

Do we demand that the only proof we will accept is that of dead bodies and sick people? If we insist that we have to have proof in the form of deaths and disease, then we are effectively condemning this generation. We are treating them like lab rats in an experiment with no controls.

With wireless radiation everywhere, there is no unexposed control group. The time for studying the effects of cell phone radiation when you could find people who were not users of phones is long gone. And that is also not an accident. We now know enough to take simple steps to reduce our exposures to keep ourselves and our families safer.

We can no longer compare those who use phones with those who do not. We must learn from the cases depicted here and from what the animals are trying to tell us.

So how are consumers to know what technology is safer? The Environmental Protection Agency sets standards for testing tailpipe emissions from cars. The National Highway Traffic Safety Administration sets crash standards for evaluating the safety of cars. Yet when it comes to testing and evaluating phones and other wireless radiating devices we are basically flying blind. Manufacturers get to select a single phone that must pass an outdated test so that millions are then sold. Only in France is there a government agency responsible for monitoring the safety of phones and other devices after they have been marketed. In August 2023, the French government halted the sales of Apple iPhone 12 due to excessive radiation. Within two weeks, Apple had issued a software update to fix that problem-- but only in France. When the Wall Street Journal reported that the iPhone 15 Pro over-heated up to 116 degrees In the United States, 'security' updates went out to fix that and other unspecified problems requiring upgrades in watches, computers and phones. In fact, you can be more sure of the safety of your microwave oven than of your wireless device.

As Professors Paul Heroux, Kent Chamberlin and others with the ICBE-EMF have shown, the technologies to craft safer devices are here and now. It is time for manufacturers to step up and produce safer devices and tell us that they have done this. Informed consumers are increasingly creating a ready market for improved devices. The government and industry should stop hiding behind the complexity of the issue and create conditions for generating and promoting safer technologies.

14

Everything You Need to Know About Safer Technology But Are Afraid to Ask

The greatest enemy of knowledge is not ignorance, it is the illusion of knowledge.

~Stephen Hawking

W e live in the age of the technological imperative where the possibility that something can be technically accomplished has been mistaken for evidence that it should be crafted. The age at which children receive their first phones or other wireless devices keeps dropping. At the same time, practical information about why and how to reduce exposures remains poorly understood. Simply put: wireless radiating devices operate by sending and receiving microwave signals that can enter bodies, brains, and the environment depending on where and how the signals are deployed. The range of devices that have gone wireless boggles the mind: breast pumps, minders that light up the carton when an egg is about to expire, water filters that automatically order their replacements, toothbrushes that allow you to see inside your mouth and record how long and well you brush, a fork that tells you when you are eating too fast, a dog

283

food dispenser that allows you to talk to your dog remotely and offer treats when it responds, a wireless cradle that rocks the crying newborn and plays mamma's soothing voice, and of course, vagina-based Bluetooth-enabled speakers.

To meet rapidly growing demands for more bandwidth to operate these inventions and enable faster-streaming games, porn, and videos, 5G wireless-emitting network antennas are popping outside of bedroom windows and alongside school buildings. Promising faster downloads to keep up with carefully cultivated appetites for the latest digital novelties promoted as essentials, one million new 5G network antennas are slated for the U.S. alone. With more than twenty two billion cell phones and wireless devices globally, there are now three times more networked digital devices than people. Thousands of apps are designed for undiscriminating and easily addicted audiences — toddlers and infants.

As the successor to 4G, 5G networks are widely advertised to yield higher-speed downloads and connectivity with little to no delay. Unsaid in the blitz for the latest and greatest tech is that for 5G networks to operate at peak modes, two things are required. First, people must purchase new 5G routers, new 5G phones, new 5G computers, etc. Second, a network must exist that seamlessly connects these devices by beam-forming between them and a mostly not-yet-ready-for-primetime network that requires 5G antennas to be placed about every football field apart throughout urban America. Thus, 5G remains a massive marketing strategy that only works with new equipment and networks. To forge these new networks, governments worldwide are being blitzed with legislative proposals blocking local control over antenna siting or consideration of the environmental impacts such a network imposes. Without any grounds for objecting to where antennas are located, urban dwellers are waking up to thirty-foot tall masts that place 5G radiating devices within feet of their bedroom windows. At the center of 5G systems sit antennas that have the theoretical capacity to send and receive messages that are wireless radiation signals from more than a thousand devices at the same time. This will also connect dog collars, dialysis pumps, blender tops, phones, and even running shoes to body-worn monitors, formerly known as wristwatches.

Yet, while information and communications technologies forge new applications — some of questionable value — scientific evidence continues to mount indicating serious physical, emotional, and psychological impacts caused by the use of cell phones and other wireless devices. We may never know why Bill Gates and Steve Jobs did not permit their own children to use many of the devices that their companies marketed. But nowadays more and more parents and teachers are waking up to the fact that over-reliance on digital technology can impair learning, growth, or development.

Arianna Huffington recommends students turn off their phones and get more sleep. Speaking with students at the University of Southern California in 2018, she said, "The goal of machines and software is to minimize downtime. But for the human operating system, downtime is not a bug; it's a feature."

Keeping devices and ourselves on at all times with no downtime has proven a brilliant marketing strategy, compounding and heightening the sense of urgency that pervades modern life. Turning all of us into emergency responders who must be on call constantly impedes personal growth and intimate relationships. This always-on mentality has also been found to undermine young children's education and speech acquisition. A growing number of schools in the U.S., France, Israel, India, and other nations now ban phones in schools or severely limit their use, to reduce detrimental impacts on learning. At the same time, more and more parents are working to reclaim family dinner table conversations by keeping all phones out of reach. Unfortunately, the pandemic unleashed a dependence on wireless technologies that many experts understand is contributing to a global decline in the mental health and cognitive performance of children and teenagers, as the World Health Organization reported.

Despite the fact that an ever increasing number of scientists and doctors caution that exposure to wireless radiation can be physically and psychologically unsafe especially for children, the U.S. Federal Communications Commission has dug in its heels. As of the drafting of this postscript, the FCC has not responded to the U.S. Court of Appeals for the D.C. Circuit mandate in *EHT et al. v the FCC, 2021* that the agency provide a reasoned review of evidence regarding children's unique vulnerability, the health impacts of long-term exposure, the ubiquity of wireless devices, and the antiquated use of the Specific Absorption Rate (SAR) metric, which models only the heating properties of wireless radiation using tests that put a space between the phone and body. The court also ordered the agency to evaluate growing numbers of scientific studies from the U.S. Fish and Wildlife Service and independent scientists showing that wireless radiation affects trees, birds, bees, and other living creatures.

In the meantime, several national governments, including Belgium, Taiwan, France, Cyprus, and Israel, have passed laws and/ or launched major efforts to reduce exposures to wireless radiation, especially for children. The figure that follows shows that legally allowable cell tower radiation limits in several countries such as Switzerland (for schools and homes), India, China, Russia, and several Eastern European countries are ten to one hundred times more restrictive than those of the U.S., Australia, and Canada.

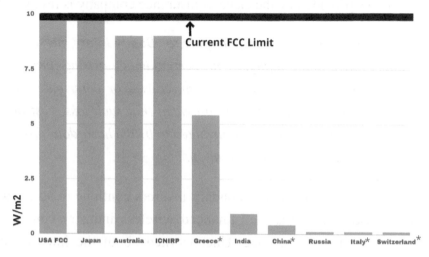

The reasons so many governments have issued more restrictive standards than the U.S. are easy to grasp. For two decades, studies submitted to the FCC docket (which can be found at FCC.gov) consistently show that legally allowed levels of wireless radiation can wield serious adverse effects on human health and the physical environment on which life depends. Recognizing these biological effects of wireless radiation, Russian and Chinese scientists were early leaders in research that formed the foundation for considerably reduced safety levels in those countries. Others, such as Switzerland and Italy, employ the precautionary principle, which calls for taking preventive action to reduce exposures despite some uncertainty regarding the underlying science.

As reported in the first edition of *Disconnect* and reiterated in the new preface to this edition, major global secondary insurers like Lloyd's of London and Swiss Re continue to refuse to provide coverage for any health or environmental damages from electromagnetic fields. They liken the financial risks to those posed by asbestos, from which damages bankrupted several firms.

The exclusions in the policy covering the Portland, Oregon, public schools provided by the Genesis insurance company is revealing:

> *"This insurance does not apply to: Bodily injury, personal injury, advertising injury, or property damage arising directly or indirectly out of, resulting from, caused or contributed to by electromagnetic radiation, provided that such loss, cost or expense results from or is contributed to by the hazardous properties of electromagnetic radiation."*

At the same time that secondary insurers continue to vote with their pocketbooks, the well-financed wireless industry continues to "war-game" the science. Unconcerned about the integrity of any studies, the industry's message becomes: health effects are not established and remain uncertain. Multi-million dollar public relations efforts fund massive promotions that manufacture doubt and provide generous political donations across political parties. The closing scenario of the movie *Thank You For Smoking* seems eerily relevant. A group of advertising experts for the MOD Squad — merchants of death, including tobacco, guns, and alcohol — is recruiting a new member to their fold. An off-camera voice questions a panel of uncomfortable-appearing men who begin squirming in their seats.

"Well, is it true? Do cellphones cause brain cancer?"

As the men all begin murmuring, the questioner interrupts.

"Gentlemen, I want you to practice saying these words in front of a mirror. 'At this time, although we are concerned about the matter, there is no *direct* evidence linking cellphones and cancer.'"

This dramatic vignette makes it clear. Raising doubt in the public mind about science remains a critical byproduct of the industry. Many well-remunerated experts have built successful businesses by raising doubts in otherwise respected publications such as *The New York Times* or *Forbes Magazine* about scientific reports that wireless radiation from cell phones and other wireless devices can have damaging impacts on human health or the environment.

"Doubt is our product," rang the motto of tobacco industry public relations experts. Just as this brilliant dark comedy movie about promoting smoking had proposed, the fomenting of questions about the quality of science on cell phones and health quickly morphed into a major strategy. Experts in the expanding field of product defense increasingly skew the scientific literature, manufacture and magnify scientific uncertainty, and influence policy decisions.

The International Commission on Non-Ionizing Radiation Protection (ICNIRP), which asserts that the sole biological impact of wireless radiation is heating, remains a widely cited source by U.S. and European authorities. However, that dominion has been rejected by a growing number of authorities, including the European Environment Agency. Many governments that have conducted their own searching review of the science adopted precautionary policies to reduce children's exposures in order to prevent harm. The errors and inaccuracies of ICNIRP that were charted in the first edition of *Disconnect* have now also been further detailed and documented by several highly respected experts, including James C. Lin, former editor-in-chief of the journal *Bioelectromagnetics*; Henry Lai, one of the founders of the field; and physician-scientist Lennart Hardell, a pioneer in public health research. They have separately detailed numerous technical inaccuracies and inherent biases found in several recent ICNIRP reports. In a critical analysis of the historical literature, Professor Lai showed that studies that tend to find no long-term chronic health effects have been published primarily by industry-sponsored scientists. In contrast, studies that indicate potential hazards to public health or the environment from wireless radiation are much more likely to be produced by scientists with independent funding.

In truth, studying the human impact of wireless radiation remains a highly contentious subject for two reasons. First, it is difficult to tease out various causal factors in evaluating chronic illnesses such as brain, thyroid, breast, or colo-rectal cancers. What people eat, where they live, how they work, and other lifestyle factors are pivotal in setting the stage for cancer. Information about such matters has never been easy to acquire in modern nations. Second, the doubt-manufacturing industry operates in high gear, sometimes raising legitimate questions about important issues but chiefly to generate skepticism about results. So long as people remain in doubt, then inaction carries the day.

Despite these considerable difficulties, studies published after the 2010 first edition of *Disconnect* find that persons who have used mobile or cordless phones for a decade or longer have significantly increased risks of brain cancer — a fact first noted by the International Agency for Research on Cancer (IARC) in 2011 and subsequently corroborated by additional reports. In 2019, a Yale University investigation of 900 people found cell phone radiation associated with doubled rates of thyroid cancer among those with specific genetic variations.

In 2018, my colleagues and I published an analysis of all the human studies that had been completed on brain cancer and cell phone use since the IARC 2011 report classified such radiation as "possibly carcinogenic to humans" — the same category as chloroform and some pesticides. We specifically rejected the so-called million-women study of menopausal women from the U.K. that found no association between reported cell phone use and brain cancer. That study of about three-quarters of a million women had asked these older women if they ever, never or, daily used cell phones. Only eighteen percent of those polled had used phones half-an-hour daily. This study yielded critically important information about hormone replacement therapy, as it was designed to do, but it was never set up to produce results regarding cell phone use. This was added onto the analysis long after the research project had been created. In our review of all relevant reports, we concluded:

> *When considered with recent animal experimental evidence, the recent epidemiological studies strengthen and support the conclusion that RFR should be categorized as carcinogenic to humans (IARC Group 1).*

In that same report, we also recommended an easy way to obtain additional information on the role of wireless radiation in human health: Cross-sectional studies that take a snapshot of health at a given time. While phones and other closely held wireless radiating devices are universal, surveys of their impact can easily divide current mobile phone users into high-, medium-, and low-use groups to report on hearing, vision, memory, reaction time, and other indicators that can be easily assessed through standardized computer-based tests.

Why are these simple cross-sectional snapshots of health not being conducted? Becasue if you don't want to know, just don't ask.

In 2022, the ICBE-EMF reached conclusions that many independent experts support:

> *"The past 25 years of extensive research on RFR demonstrates that the assumptions underlying the FCC's and ICNIRP's exposure limits are invalid and continue to present a public health harm. Adverse effects observed at exposures below the assumed threshold SAR include non-thermal induction of reactive oxygen species, DNA damage, cardiomyopathy, carcinogenicity, sperm*

damage, and neurological effects, including electromagnetic hypersensitivity. Also, multiple human studies have found statistically significant associations between RFR exposure and increased brain and thyroid cancer risk. Yet, in 2020, and in light of the body of evidence reviewed in this article, the FCC and ICNIRP reaffirmed the same limits that were established in the 1990s. Consequently, these exposure limits, which are based on false suppositions, do not adequately protect workers, children, hypersensitive individuals, and the general population from short-term or long-term RFR exposures.

In a 2023 report, members of ICBE-EMF noted that charters of professional engineering and other organizations commit to placing human safety above all other considerations. This expressed concern with social impacts of technology contrasts sharply with the lack of concerns for such consequences that undergirds policies of the wireless industry. While expanding digital capacity has radically transformed and improved many aspects of modern life, the absence of efforts to anticipate and reduce negative impacts remains a notable failure.

Engineering can contemplate many technically practical solutions aimed at reducing cell phone users' RFR exposures. Software-based solutions controlling RFR emissions, as well as hardware changes to antenna designs, should not be expensive to implement, and would only mildly influence the habits of cell phone users. Although these solutions are available, it seems that in many cases, the industry has either not implemented them, or, in some cases, has even fought exposure abatements by preventing public education about RFR exposures. ...

We firmly believe that RFR exposures to living tissues should be avoided when possible and that RFR power absorbed by the user's body is wasted and harmful to health. In all likelihood, our recommendations for cell phone alterations would improve the lifespan of both humans and batteries.

In addition, the Oceania Radiofrequency Science Advisory Association (ORSAA), an independent group of experts and professionals from South Asia, has published several studies highlighting how independent science contradicts ICNIRP's opinion that heating is the sole harm to be avoided. In sum, ORSAA and ICBE-EMF provide a much-needed perspective, questioning the technological imperative which assumes that merely because something can be accomplished, it should be undertaken and allowed to proceed. At its most extreme, this mandate has produced situations where infants and toddlers are learning to swipe before they can walk or talk, impeding and curtailing their language and physical development.

Unfortunately, the U.S. and most other governments have largely been blind to these concerns or the mounting toll on our mental health from the increasingly wireless world. They have also ignored the numerous expert advisories calling for control and reductions of wireless exposures that have been issued in the years since *Disconnect* was first published.

An explanation for the FCC's failure to take proactive steps can be found in a critical 2015 report from Harvard's Edmund J. Safra Center for Ethics by Norm Alster. Describing the FCC as a "captured agency," Alster detailed how the wireless industry has bought inordinate access to — and power over — the FCC. There is a "revolving door" between the wireless industry and government regulators as FCC commissioners move back and forth between holding government positions and wireless companies' leadership. Thus, the fox is in charge of the henhouse.

As a result, federal agencies have fast-tracked the deployment of 5G, or fifth-generation wireless technology, with no scientific foundation for this expansion. 5G and the internet of things (IoT) are put forward as urgently needed in order to connect the millions of new wirelessly connected products, including self-driving cars, smart home systems, and an array of machine-to-machine communications. What's driving the need for this faster system? Your washing machine, coffee pot, doorbell, and nannycam can all talk to and be controlled by your cell phone. These questionable utilities also enhance the capacity of hackers and thieves to know when you are at home and what you are doing.

Spurred by an effective telecom lobbying campaign, second only to pharmaceuticals in its expenditures, the FCC has moved to expedite the development of 5G and the IoT. In 2019, the FCC issued new rules to fast-track what they dubbed "small cell" deployment — another name for 5G. A "small cell" is not truly small, as it can be larger than a walk-in freezer. The term is given to the antennas needed for a 5G network to function and to escape serious regulatory review. In the telecom world, small is not merely deemed beautiful but also eludes regulatory attention. The premise is that small network antennas need not fall under regulatory scrutiny afforded to larger network equipment.

Compared to 2G and 3G network infrastructure, 5G requires many more cellular antennas. Some 5G networks operate through higher-frequency radio waves that have vast data capacity but cannot travel as far as 4G. Those higher-frequency waves also cannot as easily penetrate through trees, buildings, and other obstacles. Hence companies claim they need more and closer "small" cell antenna sites densely installed in cities. In many instances, trees are cut down to prioritize transmission of network signals. Where 4G might require 50 antennas, 5G may require up to 2,000. 5G equipment can be installed, for example, atop a short pole 10 to 30 feet tall. Some 5G arrays can contain 1,024 distinct signal-transmitting antennas. Global costs of 5G networks are estimated to run close to three-quarters of a trillion dollars with a million new antennas in the U.S. alone.

"Small cell" wireless facilities in front of homes.
These poles are topped with 5G or 4G antennas.

The FCC's 2019 rules limit the ability of state and local authorities to restrict antenna proliferation in residential areas and limit fees paid by telecoms for this access. Additional federal limits are being bandied about as this book goes to press. In addition, about half of U.S. states have passed small cell streamlining laws, which further strip the authority of local communities to decide how and where 5G and 4G cell antenna installations are located. Several pending federal laws would make it quite difficult to object to the location of any newly proposed 5G antenna.

These federal and state 5G streamlining laws are, in effect, corporate land grabs as well as marketing ploys. Telecommunications companies now have easy access to public rights-of-way across the nation. Note that in Israel, Belgium, and other high-tech nations, it would be against the law to construct such antennas near schools or hospitals. However, the U.S. government permits such installations.

TB1	Millimeter Wave Bay for Operator 1 Ultra-Fast 5G Service
TB2	Millimeter Wave Bay for Operator 2 Ultra-Fast 5G Service
TB3 * TB4	Millimeter Wave Bay or Sub 6 GHz Shared Bay for 4G LTE + 5G for additional coverage and capacity for CBRS and/or IOT to support neutral host providers and technologies
TB5	Optimized Wi-Fi structure and siting locations improve coverage and performance of free public gigabit Wi-Fi

Left image: One of the 2,000 5G towers slated for New York City,
Right image: Graphic from the New York Office
of Technology's PowerPoint on 5G towers, 2023.

With no public notice, new 5G cell network antennas are emerging in neighborhoods on street lights and utility poles, some as tall as a three-story building. These 5G antenna arrays will need to rely on 4G infrastructure to connect older devices.

It is not widely understood that most of today's 5G antennas will not immediately replace current technologies. Instead, 5G networks add more density of wireless network signals into an already packed electromagnetic environment filled with 4G frequencies and signals. 5G networks include multiple frequency ranges from the low-band, used in cell phone networks for decades, to mid-band and high-band submillimeter and millimeter wave frequencies. The industry's goal is to ensure the purchase of new 5G routers, phones, computers, baby monitors, coffee pots, dishwashers, and doorbells. Whether this will improve productivity, speed, and access remains to be seen.

Furthermore, the term 5G used in City Council meetings to sell communities on allowing corporations to erect new poles in public rights-of-way can be grossly misleading. What are being sold in the short term are simply more and more 4G wireless antennas — termed densification. Moreover, network providers do not share their toys so each neighborhood might have three to five different telecom companies grafting their networks in the same vicinity onto light poles or erecting new structures. T-Mobile, AT&T, CenturyLink, Spectrum, and Verizon must build their own networks. Each will require its own set of multi-antenna equipment, selling its own devices or linked to its partners. With numerous new wireless antenna sites on each block, the everyday levels of radio frequency emissions and exposures throughout each neighborhood will intensify in a way that has never before been undertaken in the short history of this remarkable industry.

Informed by expert scientist appeals, citizens in many countries are objecting to the explosive rollout of new 5G wireless network antennas that is taking place without widespread awareness of the established and continuing research on the impacts of radio frequency radiation on the human body, wildlife, and the environment. The International EMF Scientist Appeal to the U.N. to Protect Humans and Wildlife from Electromagnetic Fields and Wireless Technology (emfscientist.org) was launched in 2015 and as of 2023 had been signed by 257 scientists from 44 nations, all of whom have published research in the field. This appeal states:

> *Numerous recent scientific publications have shown that EMF affects living organisms at levels well below most international and national guidelines. Effects include increased cancer risk, cellular stress, increase in harmful free radicals, genetic damages, structural and functional changes of the reproductive*

system, learning and memory deficits, neurological disorders, and negative impacts on general well-being in humans. Damage goes well beyond the human race, as there is growing evidence of harmful effects to both plant and animal life.

This international expert group issued the following specific requests with which we at Environmental Health Trust agree:

1. Protect children and pregnant women.
2. Strengthen guidelines and regulatory standards.
3. Encourage manufacturers to develop safer technology.
4. Require utilities responsible for generating, transmitting, distributing, and monitoring electricity to maintain adequate power quality and ensure proper electrical wiring to minimize harmful ground currents.
5. Inform the public of the potential health risks from electromagnetic energy and teach harm reduction strategies.
6. Educate medical professionals about the biological effects of electromagnetic energy and train them to diagnose and treat patients with electromagnetic sensitivity.
7. Mandate industry cooperation with researchers and encourage governments to fund independent studies for training and research on electromagnetic fields and health.
8. Require media to disclose experts' financial relationships with the industry when citing their opinions regarding health and safety aspects of EMF-emitting technologies.
9. Establish radiation-free safe zones.

In 2017, Dr. Lennart Hardell, a prolific epidemiologist and Professor Emeritus of Medicine in Sweden, launched the 5G Appeal (www.5gappeal.eu), calling for the European Union to halt the rollout of 5G. Signed by more than 430 scientists and doctors, that document declares:

Scientists and doctors call for a moratorium on the roll-out of 5G. 5G will substantially increase exposure to radio frequency electromagnetic fields, RF-EMF, that has been proven to be harmful for humans and the environment.

Numerous other international groups have issued similar appeals. As just one example, in 2018, the International Society of Doctors for the Environment reviewed the evidence on the matter and took this position on 5G:

Evidence is growing that exposure to frequencies over 30GHz — planned for 5G — could alter gene expression, increase the temperature of the skin, stimulate cell proliferation, alter the functions of cell membrane and neuro-muscular systems, and are able to modulate the synthesis of proteins involved in inflammatory and immunologic processes, with possible systemic effects.

Environmental Health Trust has compiled these and other appeals on its website, ehtrust.org.

At this point in time the science is clear. We know that current regulatory limits — set solely to avoid the short-term effect of heating — are not protective of human health, wildlife, or the general environment. Exposures must be substantially reduced and safer alternatives used whenever possible, preferring wired rather than wireless systems following the practical advice noted below and more details on our website.

California's Right-to-Know Law

Citizen efforts to promote sensible policies have evolved in parallel to the scientific efforts noted above. For several years,

Ellie Marks served as director of government and public affairs for EHT. Testifying before the U.S. Congress and working diligently with California State Representatives, Ellie became a magnet for families with cell phone-related cancers. Many of their heartrending stories can be found on the EHT website as cell phone survivors and non-survivors.

After *Disconnect* was published in 2010, Ellie and then-EHT board member attorney Harry Lehman proved unrelenting and unstoppable in helping those contending with cell phone-related injuries, illnesses, and deaths. With their support EHT worked alongside other organizations and California residents to persuade then-Mayor of San Francisco Gavin Newsom and the entire San Francisco Board of Supervisors to pass the Cell Phone Right-to-Know Law in 2010, requiring that cell phones were labeled for their radiation levels (Specific Absorption Rates) at point of sale. The law was updated in 2011 by unanimous vote. As you can see in the following image, the San Francisco Department of Environment developed educational posters and fact sheets that explained how cell phones emitted radio frequency radiation and detailed simple ways consumers can minimize their exposure. The information was to be posted in retail stores so that people were informed when they went shopping for cell phones.

It was a good idea then and it remains a good idea now. The heroic struggles on behalf of that law are now legendary. The Cellular Telephone Industries Association (CTIA) immediately sued the city demanding the law be overturned because it violated the companies' free speech rights. The CTIA said the ordinance would cause confusion and mislead consumers. "The FCC has determined that all wireless phones legally sold in the United States are 'safe,'" CTIA spokesman John Walls said in a CTIA press release.

As the legal battle dragged on, the industry threatened the city with having to pay the industry's top-dollar multi-million-dollar legal costs if it prevailed. Deputy City Attorney C. Vincent Chhabria determined that the city could not afford the risk that a reviewing judge might agree that requiring the posting of notices about cell phone radiation and the need to take precautions with children constituted a form of "compelled speech." In the end, the city agreed not to enforce its own law to get out from under this draconian prospect of paying millions for industry lawyers.

Chhabria now sits as a judge for the Northern District of California.

Taking its cue from San Francisco's effort to inform people about the fine print warnings now buried within cell phone operating systems, in 2015, the City of Berkeley, California, adopted a law crafted with the help of Harvard Law Professor Lawrence Lessig. The law's wording seemed straightforward at the time and has proved prophetic regarding science. The law called for a poster warning at the point of sale:

THE CITY OF BERKELEY REQUIRES THAT YOU BE PROVIDED THE FOLLOWING NOTICE:

"To assure safety, the Federal Government requires that cell phones meet radio frequency (RF) exposure guidelines. If you carry or use your phone in a pants or shirt pocket or tucked into a bra when the phone is ON and connected to a wireless network, you may exceed the federal guidelines for exposure to RF radiation. ~~This potential risk is greater for children.~~*

Refer to the instructions in your phone or user manual for information about how to use your phone safely."

* This statement was removed from the original ordinance after legal challenges.

When the industry challenged the legality of this notice in the Northern District of California Court, Judge Edward M. Chen sided with it. The judge determined that Berkeley was "overwarning" with its requirement that people be notified that phones are tested at some distance from the phantom body of a large, tall male and should not be kept on the body and that children required special considerations.

With remarkable bureaucratic arrogance, the FCC complained that requiring that people be informed about testing distances and limits could impair the capacity of the industry to develop and grow. According to the FCC, the Berkeley Right-to-Know Law interfered with federal oversight of the telecom industry because that ordinance "overwarns" consumers. The FCC claimed that it was doing an adequate job of educating consumers about safe cell phone use, although it did not provide a single instance of that effort.

George Orwell could not have written a better script: it's okay for phones to be tested away from the big, male body and at some distance from the brain. But it's not okay to tell people that this is the case. Nor is it okay to tell people that if they or their children keep phones directly on the body, they exceed the 1996 standards developed to avoid heating a big, male dummy during a six-minute call.

Dr. Joel Moskowitz of the School of Public Health, University of California, Berkeley successfully sued the State of California to release these records, including all the specific drafts of public education materials advising people about why and how to use phones safely. His website provides a running digital archival record of these and other pertinent developments and details the hypocrisy of the matter.

In overturning the Berkeley law, Judge Chen bluntly stated, "The FCC is tasked with balancing the competing objectives of ensuring public health and safety and promoting the development and growth of the telecommunications network and related services."

Moskowitz noted that although Berkeley could have appealed the ruling, it decided to settle the case with the CTIA by agreeing not to enforce the "right-to-know" ordinance that had been in effect since 2016. In return, the CTIA agreed not to seek attorneys' fees. Professor Lessig, who served as the lead attorney for the city in this case, proposed that since the right-to-know ordinance "remains on the books awaiting a better FCC ... We should get through this crisis and then see what makes the most sense."

At this juncture, my colleagues and I at EHT and around the world believe we have amassed sufficient new information that it now makes "sense" to undertake a major public educational campaign to promote the Right-to-Know Law at local levels.

Given the tragedies that fill our screens today, this may seem an inopportune moment to raise concerns that a vital technology on which so many depend can fundamentally compromise our health and well-being. But we cannot afford the luxury of waiting for a better, later time to bring attention to the physical, psychological, and spiritual toll of wireless radiating devices, especially for the billions of young children who are living in a sea of radiation. We have no choice but to demand safer hardware and software now.

We hope that the materials in this book and on our website provide ample grounds to ensure that people are fully informed about why and how to use technology more safely. We believe that current circumstances for phones are like those that existed for airbags and seatbelts for cars in the 1960s. Evidence of harm is real. Ways to reduce that harm are clear. It is time for industry and government to produce safer technology, building upon existing patents that can reduce radiation. In the meantime, please share this new updated edition with all those whose brains and bodies you care about.

Remember, there once was a time when smoking on airplanes and in the environments of young children was perfectly legal. As a young scientist, I worked with others to establish that what was commonplace then endangered public health for years to come. The case for precaution regarding wireless radiation is abundantly clear. What's lacking is the political courage to protect us and the world in which we live from this avoidable environmental hazard.

How many more must die before we do the right thing?

15

HOW TO PROTECT YOURSELF, YOUR FAMILY, AND YOUR COMMUNITY

By Theodora Scarato, MSW,
Executive Director of Environmental Health Trust

I. How To Protect Yourself And Your Family

Today's homes are filled with an ever growing number of microwave-RF frequency emitting devices from tablets to laptops, Wi-Fi toys, and all types of "smart" things. These include AirPods, which are Class 3 Bluetooth emitting devices that have never been tested for safety and can transmit radio frequency radiation to and through young developing brains and eyes. Children face a lifetime of microwave radiation exposures that increase risks for cancer, reproductive damage, and numerous other health impacts. Furthermore, children and the rest of us are also becoming psychologically and physiologically addicted to the dopamine hit caused by interactive screen use.

Fortunately, the AAP continues to recommend reducing wireless radiation exposure, particularly among young children. More than a dozen countries have policies to minimize the use of cell phones by children. Their government public health agencies advise on various ways to minimize wireless exposures to the brain, including recommendations to use speakerphones or text messaging — instead of voice calls using wireless earpieces or a cell phone held up next to the head.

As Dr. Davis has discussed throughout this book, government action in the United States and elsewhere is lacking. Instead of waiting for government action, here is what you can do right now to help keep you and your family safe:

Reduce Your Exposure

Anything that uses cellular, Wi-Fi, or Bluetooth emits wireless radiation. You can start to reduce your exposure by taking an inventory of wireless sources at home, work, and school. You may be surprised how many items you own emit wireless radiation: cell phones, wireless headphones, wireless routers, tablets, laptops, computers, wireless printers, wireless keyboards and mice, signal boosters, cordless phones, Bluetooth speakers, gaming consoles, wireless wearables like watches and rings, digital assistants like Siri and Alexa, wireless doorbells, wireless thermostats, and many other "smart" devices. Most new appliances are among those "smart" devices as they come with radiating components that enable them to wirelessly connect to the internet. These radiation-emitting components in appliances are sometimes complicated to turn off but it can be done.

Here are three key ways to decrease your exposure:

1. **Reduce the amount of time you spend on cell phones and wireless-enabled devices.** Learn how to set devices to airplane mode to minimize RF radiation emissions.

2. **Increase your distance from wireless devices.** Wireless phones should not be held next to the head or body. Laptops and tablets should not be on laps.

3. **Replace wireless technology with safer alternatives.** You can quickly reduce your daily exposure by getting into the

habit of using corded landline or ethernet connections for voice calls and internet whenever possible. Swapping out wireless tools for corded models is easier than you think.

Measure Wireless Emissions

It helps to know the levels of RF you are exposed to daily. You need a meter that detects and measures wireless radiation because you cannot always perceive wireless radiation with your senses.

Some of the newest phone models on the market continue to transmit (to allow geolocating a lost phone) even when fully powered off. We recommend you use a meter to test phone models.

Some local libraries, with persuasion from communities and citizens' groups, have purchased radio frequency meters that you can borrow just as you would borrow books. EHT has developed a library grant plan and provides RF-meter recommendations on its website, ehtrust.org.

Using a borrowed meter, you can identify sources of radiation in your environment.

Using Airplane Mode and Other Settings to Stop Wireless Emissions

Just like cell phones, all wireless devices (such as the home cordless phone bases, gaming consoles, Wi-Fi speakers, routers, and printers) emit wireless radiation non-stop — even when not actively being used. Having a meter to measure the radio frequency emissions can help you determine the emitting antennas in each device are off or on.

There are two ways to stop a wireless cell phone from emitting wireless radiation. The first way is to power off the cell phone and fully disconnect it from electricity. The other way is to go to settings, turn on airplane mode, and check that all of the cell phone's wireless antennas are off — including, including Bluetooth, Hotspots, Wi-Fi, location tracking, 4G, 5G, and others. It used to be that turning on

Airplane mode took care of this all in one step, but many new cell phone models have multiple antennas, therefore you need to check all of them in settings.

You can also set shortcuts on your computer to turn on airplane mode and turn off all antennas.

Best Practices for All Your Devices

The following recommendations will help you reduce your radiation exposure from wireless devices.

Cell Phones

Cell phones should be kept away from the head and body. Do not use or hold a cell phone close to your abdomen or next to your child. Cell phones are not toys and should not be used as pacifiers or distractions for children. When you hand a child a phone or tablet, ensure it is on airplane mode and all wireless antennas are toggled off. Bring a toy to the grocery store instead of handing your child a phone.

You can minimize wireless and Wi-Fi use by selecting safer connections like corded phones and cabled internet. Here are other simple ways you can reduce exposure:

- Use a speakerphone instead of holding the phone to your head.
- Do not sleep with a cell phone on or near you.
- Use a battery-powered alarm clock rather than your phone's alarm.
- Do not carry a cell phone in your pocket.
- Do not carry a cell phone tucked into your bra, pants, or head-wear.
- Choose to text instead of making voice or video calls.
- Text with your cell phone at a distance from your body instead of close to your chest.
- Close apps you are not using and turn off background refresh

for apps that don't need it. Every time an app refreshes, the phone connects to the internet, creating firsthand and second-hand wireless exposures whether or not you are actively using the phone.

- Turn off antennas you are not using, such as Bluetooth, Cellular, Hotspot, Data, 4G, 5G, etc.
- Choose a wired air tube headset instead of wireless headphones.
- Choose a corded landline at home and work instead of a cell phone.
- Set your phone to airplane mode, and turn off Wi-Fi/Bluetooth/Cellular more often.
- Connect your cell phone to the internet via an ethernet cable and turn off all wireless antennas. Connection via ethernet allows you to do everything on the phone you would do on Wi-Fi. All you need is a special adapter. See more details at ehtrust.org and healthytechhome.org.

Beware: Cell phones increase RF emissions in some settings

A cell phone will increase its wireless RF output in certain situations. Reduce use in these circumstances:

- Low service areas: If one or two bars are displayed, the cell phone will emit more energy because it must work harder to connect with the network base station (cell tower or Wi-Fi router). Turn antennas off in these situations.
- Moving large files: Streaming audio, video or sending and receiving large files increases wireless emissions. To watch movies or listen to podcasts and music playlists on your phone, download them first, then turn off Wi-Fi and other wireless antennas and switch to airplane mode before watching or listening.

- Metal surroundings: RF often increases inside cars, buses, subways, and elevators. Turn off antennas to stop emissions inside vehicles.

Computers and Tablets
- Devices should rest on a table not on your lap.
- Turn off Wi-Fi antennas whenever you are not actively using Wi-Fi. Also, turn off Bluetooth and other antennas when not in use.
- If you are in a situation where you must use Wi-Fi, maximize the distance between your body and the device (computer, tablet, Wi-Fi router, etc.).
- Pre-download movies and games and choose applications that can be used offline so that you can turn the Wi-Fi off. This way, when you or a child uses the app, the wireless antennas are not radiating.
- Sync word processing and other software programs at a time you manually choose. This way you can work with wireless antennas off and sync to the cloud later when you are not close to the syncing devices.
- Eliminate exposure 100 percent by connecting computers to the internet with an ethernet cable instead of Wi-Fi. After you connect with ethernet, remember to turn off the Wi-Fi and Bluetooth in your computer's settings.
- Use wired and corded accessories and peripherals instead of Wi-Fi or Bluetooth for keyboards, mice, speakers, printers, headphones, etc.
- Forward text notifications from your phone to your computer. This way, you can still text but without the RF exposure. Go to healthytechhome.org to learn more.
- Use blue-light blocking glasses, especially in the evenings. Blue light interferes with the natural production of melatonin,

a natural antioxidant and hormone that plays a vital role in inducing and regulating sleep.

Home and Office Phones

Cordless phones use the same type of wireless radiation as cell phones. The phone-charging bases are like mini cell tower base stations in your home, emitting wireless radiation 24/7 even when no one is using the phone.

- Install a corded phone (not cordless) in your home and workplace.
- Keep your landline active. That's the best choice for phone calls.
- If you do not have a separate landline, consider a VoIP or internet phone option. This type of equipment can connect to a corded phone.
- Run phone cables to all rooms where you need a phone.
- Forward your cell phone to your non-wireless phone to minimize cell phone use.
- Buy a longer handset cord for your corded phone so you can move around the room.

Wi-Fi Internet Routers

Wi-Fi routers emit wireless radiation nonstop, even when no one is using the internet. Ensure the wireless router or modem is not located in areas where you spend a lot of time, such as the bedroom, playroom, or living room.

- Set up a 100 percent wired (instead of Wi-Fi) internet connection by plugging ethernet cables into devices. You may need adaptors easily purchased online.
- If you must have Wi-Fi, get a non-wireless modem and add a Wi-Fi router with an on/off button. You can reduce daily exposure by turning Wi-Fi off at bedtime and when not in use. Some routers are "on demand," meaning they only emit radiation when in use.

- Be aware that as long as a Wi-Fi router is on, it transmits wireless radiation.
- Do not sleep in a room with a Wi-Fi router near your bed or baby's crib.
- Do not put Wi-Fi routers in the living room, office, sleep, play areas, or rooms where you spend a lot of time.

Environmental Health Trust recommends you consider setting up ethernet connections to connect to the internet at home whenever possible. Learn more, including step-by-step instructions, at EHT's website, healthytechhome.org

Printers

Unless a wireless printer is disconnected from power, it emits wireless radiation nonstop, even when you are not using it. Thankfully, in most models, you can turn the wireless antennas off. Read the manual or contact the manufacturer.

- Connect the printer to your computer with a USB cable (not Wi-Fi) whenever possible.
- Turn the printer's Wi-Fi and Bluetooth settings off as often as possible.
- If you must use a wireless printer, unplug it when not in use or turn off antennas after each use.
- Before purchasing a printer, check that the printer has a convenient option to turn off the wireless antennas.

Wireless Wearables

"Smart" watches and fitness trackers emit wireless radiation.

- Turn off Wi-Fi, Bluetooth, and cellular while wearing the device. When you are not wearing it later, connect to transfer data.
- Purchase wearables that have airplane mode.

- Consider a non-wireless watch or fitness tracker.

Baby Monitors

Wireless baby monitors emit wireless radiation continuously when they are turned on.

- Do not place wireless monitors near cribs or children.
- Power off monitors when not in use.
- Replace wireless baby monitors with hardwired systems that use ethernet-connected security equipment.

If you are pregnant, you can reduce exposures to protect your baby.

- Keep your cell phone and other wireless devices and electronics away from your abdomen.
- Power off your phone when carrying it on your body.
- Minimize wireless and cell phone calls.
- Prefer a corded phone for voice and video calls.
- Do not set your laptop on your lap; use a table or desk.
- Do not use wireless wearables (watches, trackers, rings, etc.)
- Minimize exposure to Wi-Fi by using ethernet connections in your home.

Smart Speakers

"Smart" speakers, virtual assistants, and "smart" hubs emit wireless radiation nonstop to connect to the Wi-Fi router in your home. Be aware that "smart" speakers often have a fine print warning about putting distance between the speakers and people. We do not recommend smart speakers because most do not offer the ability to connect with ethernet. Use corded computer speakers to stream music.

Smart Meters

Nationwide, utility meters are being updated to "smart meters" that emit wireless radiation. If you already have a smart meter, contact your utility company to replace your smart meter with an analog meter. Not all smart meters emit radiation constantly; some meters only emit when a utility truck drives by it.

For those who do not yet have a smart meters, here are some options:

- Opt out on "smart" meters for electric, gas, and water if your utility allows. You might have to pay a fee to opt-out.
- Contact your elected officials in states where opting out is not available.
- Be aware of plans to convert to wireless "smart" meters in your community. Many communities have groups advocating for safer meter options. Search online for "smart meter" or "safe technology" groups in your city or state to learn more.
- Ensure your bed, couch, or other frequently used spot is not against a wall with a utility meter on the other side.
- Discuss with your neighbors the need to reduce direct exposure through shared bedroom walls.

To recap: Replace wireless with safer alternatives

- Connect your computer with ethernet instead of Wi-Fi.
- Use wired and corded (not wireless) accessories for keyboards, mice, speakers, and earbuds.
- Learn how to connect your cell phone to the internet via an ethernet cable with an adapter. After you connect via ethernet, remember to go to settings to turn off your phone's Wi-Fi and Bluetooth.
- Connect your printer with wires whenever possible.

Take a Daily Digital Detox

Technology can be lifesaving, but there are times to unplug. You can reduce exposure throughout the day by disconnecting while in several locations.

DID YOU KNOW...

ENVIRONMENTAL HEALTH TRUST

CELL PHONE RADIATION ZAPS YOUR SLEEP.

Research indicates that cell phone radiation alters brain waves during sleep.

Solution: Keep all cell phones, wireless devices, and electronics out of the bedroom. Go screen free at least an hour before bedtime.

EHTrust.org
#PracticeSafeTech

In the Bedroom

It is essential to sleep in darkness to set the body's natural clock. Avoid using digital devices in the hour before sleeping, and create a sleep sanctuary. These habits will allow for better quality of sleep and more restful sleep.

- Remove cell phones, screens, electronics, and wireless devices (including wireless speakers) from the bedroom.
- Power off Wi-Fi routers and other wireless systems before bedtime. Some people use a power strip or timer.
- Ensure the bed or crib is not near a wall with an electrical panel, large appliance, or utility meter on the other side.
- Decrease artificial light in the bedroom and invest in light-blocking curtains so the room is as dark as possible when you sleep.

315

In the Car

As a car travels, cell phones inside connect to each new cell tower the vehicle passes. Since cars are made of metal, the wireless radiation can be reflected back and forth inside the vehicle, increasing every occupant's exposure.

Here's how you can limit wireless exposure while in the car:

- Power off all cell phones and wireless devices.
- Disable any wireless antennas you can in the car's technical systems. Contact the manufacturer if necessary.
- If you are on a long car ride and your children need entertainment, use pre-downloaded movies and music instead of streaming.
- Do not use a cell phone while you are driving. Remember, most states require hands-free devices and ban texting while driving. If you must use your cell phone while in a car, distance it from your body, ensure that all other devices are off or on airplane mode, and keep calls short.

You do not need all the cell phone antennas transmitting if you need to navigate. There are two ways to get directions:

- Before driving the car, put the address into your phone so the directions for your route come up. Then turn the phone on to airplane mode. Most phones will still navigate in this mode.
- Purchase a GPS navigation model that does not have Bluetooth or cellular. Keep it in the car; always ready to go.

Want to learn more? Please visit ehtrust.org and sign up for our newsletter. EHT also has a website dedicated to educating families about reducing wireless exposure at home. Go to healthytechhome. org for step-by-step instructions on how to reduce exposure.

II. How To Get Involved To Help Reduce Everyone's Exposure

At Environmental Health Trust, our regulatory accountability and public outreach teams create digital materials that can be shared and distributed from our website. These educational materials can be easily downloaded to print yourself or at your printshop.

Here's what you can do in the public square to protect yourself and your neighbors:

Talk to Your Elected Officials

Local, state, and federal policymakers must hear from their constituents. Strong grassroots support is vital to compelling local officials to address the health and environmental issues related to cell phone radiation. Solving this issue requires federal oversight and accountability. However, most officials are not even aware of the issue.

Now is the time for constituents to contact and educate elected officials about the issues. In this way, you can inspire officials to develop protective policies. EHT has action alerts with online letter-writing campaigns so you can quickly send emails.

We recommend calling your lawmakers to schedule a meeting to request action on this issue. You can share numerous policy resources and factsheets available online at ehtrust.org with your government officials. For example, the New Hampshire State 5G Commission released a final report on its year-long investigation into the health and environmental impacts of 5G and made 15 recommendations to strengthen protective policies. Your officials need to know about this.

Ensure Your Community Has A Strong Local Wireless Ordinance

People have power. Communities can come together to develop strong local ordinances and/or zoning laws to control the proliferation of 5G, "small" cells, cell towers, or other wireless networks.

A few examples of key elements of a strong local ordinance include:

- Large setbacks between cell network antennas and homes, schools and daycares, playgrounds, sports fields, parks, hospitals, historic areas, religious institutions, and ecologically sensitive areas — noting that all those are disfavored locations for cell network equipment installations.
- Proof of compliance with the National Environmental Policy Act and Americans with Disabilities Act.
- Requirements that the applicant prove a significant gap in coverage before placing antennas close to where people live, work, and play (i.e., the disfavored locations listed above).
- Requirements for least-intrusive methods to fill any gaps, giving preference to non-wireless connectivity wherever possible (i.e. corded internet connections to homes, school, and businesses).
- Pre-and post-installation radio frequency radiation measurements.
- Adequate fall zones for poles.
- Tree protections, such as restrictions of equipment in the drip line of trees.

Even in states that have passed 5G streamlining laws, numerous other issues can be addressed with well-considered ordinances. EHT has several resources online that you can print off and share with elected and appointed officials. Physicians for Safe Technology also has resources such as Key Elements of a Strong Local Wireless Facilities Ordinance.

Raise Awareness In Your Community

Just as officials are largely unaware of the issues, so are many neighbors and friends.

Increasing awareness means getting involved. Here are a few examples of how to get the conversation started.

- Use your three minutes: Register to speak during public comment periods at your local county/city/town/village council meeting or school board meeting and share this information.

- Host a booth at your local community fair, farmers market, or PTA event.
- Organize a meeting at your library or contact local clubs like the Rotary, Lions, and Junior League to share information.
- Write letters to the editor or short posts in local newsletters or papers.
- Screen a movie or film at the local library or school. Go to ehtrust.org for film recommendations.

Demand Safer Schools

Children deserve a healthy learning environment. However, Wi-Fi networks and cell phones in classrooms are increasing unnecessary wireless radiation exposure to children. Safer solutions exist that allow internet connectivity without excessive wireless exposure.

Many schools in the U.S. and worldwide are replacing wireless with safer wired technology due to research indicating harmful effects. Internationally, France, Israel, and regions in Belgium have banned Wi-Fi in daycares and kindergartens, and officially recommend wired (instead of Wi-Fi) internet connections in classrooms.

Teacher unions are passing resolutions calling for safer technology. Parents are bringing this issue to the attention of administrators. For example, the United Educators of San Francisco passed a resolution to inform students and staff about why and how to reduce cell phone radiation. The New York State United Teachers Union also passed a resolution demanding safer technology.

In 2017, the Maryland State Children's Environmental Health And Protection Council issued the first-ever U.S. state expert organization recommendations to reduce classroom wireless exposure. The New Hampshire Commission on 5G followed a few years later, recommending that school Wi-Fi be replaced with wired networks.

In 2023 the Santa Clara County Medical Association issued Technology in School Best Practices with recommendations that includes:

- Creating a"Safe Tech" in Schools Program" to educate students and staff on why and how to reduce wireless.
- Educate school nurses on RF and blue light effects and create a monitoring and reporting program.
- Cell phone-free policies
- Take measures to RF in classroom via preferring hardwired LAN and turning off and increasing distance from Wi-Fi outers.
- Professional RF measurements
- Avoid smart meters
- Consider policy to restrict cell towers on or near school property.

Low-EMF Best Practices For Schools
- Tablets and laptops should always be on tables, not laps.
- Personal cell phones and devices should be powered off, or at least set to airplane mode, with Wi-Fi and other wireless capabilities set to OFF.
- Install wired rather than wireless LAN and communication services.
- Purchase and use computers, tablets, and other school and personal technology devices that can be ethernet-connected.
- Install computer stations and ethernet ports throughout schools for convenient internet access.
- Connect all technology devices with hardwired or plug-in cables, cords, and adapters. This includes peripherals and fixtures such as printers, projectors, scoreboard controls, boards, payment devices, landline phones, HVAC and other indoor and outdoor monitoring/control systems; network rout-

ers and other network hubs; school equipment and personal devices; computer accessories such as audio speakers, mouse, keyboard, microphone, headphones, etc. Install corded telephones in every room and common area so students and staff can communicate without cell phones. Do not install cordless phones. Replace existing cordless phones with corded alternatives.

- Install wired security systems and building technologies.
- Install wired charging systems instead of wireless charging systems for Chromebooks and other battery-powered devices.
- Ensure cell towers and 5G/4G antennas are not located on, in, or near school property.
- Teach students and staff how to reduce exposure to cell phone and wireless radiation via educational curriculum and routine staff and community education and reminders.

Recognizing that many schools may be unable or unwilling to switch from Wi-Fi to ethernet, we offer some measures for teachers and students to reduce overall wireless exposure.

- Turn off antennas whenever they are not actively being used. Devices have multiple antennas for cellular, Bluetooth, personal assistants (e.g., Siri), location, Wi-Fi, and mobile hotspot. However, users generally are only actively on the internet (via Wi-Fi). Learn how to turn on only the specific antenna needed, and always ensure all other antennas are set to off.
- Minimize streaming video; instead, pre-download videos before selecting play.
- Prefer applications that are pre-loaded and work in airplane mode. For example, cloud-based word processing programs can work offline and be synced later.

- Temporarily turn off routers and access points whenever they are not being used. Use or install an accessible power switch to manually turn off wireless transmitters whenever they are not in use.
- Reduce the transmit power of routers and access points. Generally, commercial Wi-Fi routers in schools have more powerful radiation emissions than routers consumers use at home. School routers are often excessively powered for classroom needs. TechSafeSchools explains ways that IT staff can reduce radiation emissions without affecting connectivity. Staff can:
  - Reduce the transmit power to 25 percent or less on wireless access points.
  - When the wireless access point can produce more than one radio signal (2.4GHz, 5GHz, 6GHz, or any higher GHz), enable only one radio frequency, disabling the other(s).
  - Change beacon signal interval time from 100ms to 1000ms.
  - Set routers to sleep when not in use for 10 minutes.

Educational Curriculum for Students

EHT collaborated with the Massachusetts Breast Cancer Coalition Education on educational modules to educate high school, middle school, and elementary students about reducing cell phones and other wireless radiation. The educational resources include a brief summary of the issue and what students can do to prevent exposure. Go to mbcc.org and click on the "Let's Talk Prevention" tab to download Module 3 on cell phone radiation.

Additional Resources For Schools

- The Collaborative for High-Performance Schools developed Low EMF Criteria for classrooms, including ways schools can reduce magnetic field and wireless radiation exposure.
- The New Jersey Education Association has an overview with

recommendations entitled "Minimize health risks from electronic devices."

- The journal *Building and Environment* published an article "Building science and radio frequency radiation: What makes smart and healthy buildings," which details ways to reduce EMFs in buildings.
- Techsafeschools.org has legal, technical, and scientific resources for schools.

All of these resources are available at ehtrust.org. EHT has a Wi-Fi in Schools Toolkit with shareable resources for educating school boards and parent-teacher organizations. The Toolkit includes scientific resources, a checklist to reduce EMF in classrooms and dormitories, and a briefing on wireless in the classroom.

III. The Need For Government Accountability

Currently, U.S. regulations to protect the public from the health effects of wireless devices and networks are essentially non-existent. Wireless technologies are brought to market without any testing before marketing or any surveillance afterward regarding their potential impacts on public health or the environment. Furthermore, no federal agency with health expertise is monitoring and evaluating the totality of scientific research underpinning the FCC's 1996 human exposure guidelines for cell towers and cell phones. In other words, no one is minding the store.

Unlike numerous other countries, the U.S. does not have an environmental monitoring program to measure real-world EMF levels. There is no agency that provides oversight to ensure compliance regarding RF-emission limits for towers and base stations. There is no countrywide registry or database revealing the locations of all wireless antenna installations such as "small" short cell towers or building-mounted antennas.

Federal agencies we might expect to be involved (such as the Environmental Protection Agency, the Centers for Disease Control and Prevention, the Department of Labor, the Fish and Wildlife Service, and the National Cancer Institute) have no experts on staff nor funded programs to evaluate the science. Most importantly, none of these agencies has ever released a public report or document that assesses and/or quantifies health risk or evaluates FCC limits taking into consideration the full available scientific knowledge.

The Food and Drug Administration's webpage on the issue contains numerous inaccuracies and outdated statements. In letters to lawmakers in 2019, the FDA asserted the importance of considering "the totality" of the science. Yet the agency has never reviewed all scientific research. Instead, the FDA only released an outdated, highly-skewed literature review on studies related to cancer and cell phones in 2020. The author of this FDA report remains anonymous, nor were any federal reviewers named. The FDA did not respond to letters from EHT and several scientists who wrote the FDA with questions and corrections. The FDA wrote EHT that the report was "just a literature review" in regard to the question of authorship.

The bottom line is that the FDA has never evaluated the totality of science to ensure adequate U.S. human wireless exposure limits. Such a review would include 5G technology, cell tower radiation, impacts on children, and non-cancer biological and health effects such as brain and sperm damage. No such review or risk assessment exists. Not by the FDA or any other U.S. agency.

Much of the public and U.S. elected officials seem to have fallen for the illusion that U.S. health agencies have somehow, somewhere, previously ensured the safety of cell phones and 5G networks. Wireless companies promote this myth in their propaganda. To date, federal agencies are unwilling or unable to clarify why they are not engaged in wireless radiation activities.

A study by Huss et al (2007) found that industry-funded studies were significantly less likely to report a statistically significant result. These findings have been repeated over the years. Henry Lai, an emeritus professor of bioengineering at the University of Washington, has compiled a database of peer-reviewed studies published since 1990 investigating biological effects from wireless-radiation exposure. The 2015 Harvard Press Book "Captured Agency" featured his analysis whereby he divided the studies between those that were industry-funded and those that were independently funded. He found industry-funded research identified biological effects in just 28% of studies. But 67% of non-industry funded studies found biological effects.

A 2023 analysis by scientists of the Oceania Radiofrequency Scientific Advisory Association found industry funded studies on the effects of millimeter waves also produced a lower overall proportion of "Effect" outcomes, compared to government-funded and institution-based studies.

In addition, the majority of scientific studies have found effects. In literature up to November 12, 2021. Lai tallied up the effects versus no effects for various areas of research.

- seventy-four percent found neurological effects
- ninety-two percent found oxidative effects
- sixty-seven percent found genetic effects.

In addition to health effects on humans, there are critical regulatory gaps regarding the impacts of wireless radiation on the totality of the physical environment. RF exposure limits are not designed to protect wildlife, despite urging from former senior scientist Albert Manville of the Fish and Wildlife Service that they do so. Environmental agencies do not gather data regularly to measure impacts on flora and fauna.

EHT et al. v the FCC: A Landmark Federal Court Case

In December 2019, the FCC decided there was no need to update its 1996 safety limits regarding allowable RF exposures from cell phones and towers. Despite rapid technological changes and changes in the way people use their devices in the 21st century, the FCC claimed that heat-based Specific Absorption Rate (SAR) based guidelines were adequately protective. The agency also decided that its premarket cell phone radiation test regime was adequate to show compliance with its 20th-century rules. That regime allows a distance between the phone and the human body during RF exposure testing for cell phones, which does not represent the body-contact habits of cell phone users today.

Since 2013, EHT and numerous other scientists, organizations, public health experts, and individuals have submitted extensive scientific evidence to the FCC documenting that health and environmental impacts occur at RF levels far below FCC's maximum limits. The FCC's 2019 decision was astonishing considering the overwhelming science submitted into the record for review.

Among the thousands of submissions in the FCC record, the American Academy of Pediatrics submitted a letter in 2013 requesting an update to protect children that reflects real-world use patterns. The letter stated in part:

> *Current FCC standards do not account for the unique vulnerability and use patterns specific to pregnant women and children. It is essential that any new standard for cell phones or other wireless devices be based on protecting the youngest and most vulnerable populations to ensure they are safeguarded throughout their lifetimes.*

A 2014 letter from the Department of Interior to the National Telecommunications and Information Administration was also submitted to the FCC record. It detailed the science on cell tower radiation and birds, stating:

...the electromagnetic radiation standards used by the Federal Communications Commission (FCC) continue to be based on thermal heating, a criterion now nearly 30 years out of date and inapplicable today.

There is a growing level of anecdotal evidence linking the effects of non-thermal, non-ionizing electromagnetic radiation from communication towers on nesting and roosting wild birds and other wildlife. ... Third-party peer-reviewed studies need to be conducted in the U.S. to begin examining the effects from radiation on migratory birds and other trust species.

However, in the FCC's 2019 refusal to update regulations on wireless radiation, neither these letters nor the critical wildlife issues they raised were mentioned. Numerous medical and scientific experts had recommended more protective policy. The FCC failed to mention any of them when the agency explained why it was leaving its 1996 regulations as is. It was obvious that the FCC had not taken the "hard look" nor carried out serious examination of the evidence as it claimed to have done.

The FCC's failure to provide a rationale for its decision to retain standards from 1996 to 2019 created an unprecedented opportunity to take legal action. EHT and others filed lawsuits against the FCC in 2020. These cases were consolidated before the U.S. Court of Appeals for the D.C. Circuit.

On August 13, 2021, the court ruled that the FCC's decision to keep its 1996 standards was "arbitrary and capricious." The judges found that the FCC had not adequately explained how it reached its conclusion to maintain its so-called "safety limits." The court found the FCC had ignored science submitted to them on children's vulnerability, long-term exposures, non-cancerous biological impacts, and environmental impacts, not to mention the ubiquity of wireless devices, 25 years of technological developments, and hundreds of testimonials submitted by people reporting personal injuries from exposures to wireless radiation.

The court ordered the FCC to provide a "reasoned explanation" for its decision and address the science it had ignored, specifically it mandated that the FCC:

"(i) provide a reasoned explanation for its decision to retain its testing procedures for determining whether cell phones and other portable electronic devices comply with its guidelines,

(ii) address the impacts of RF radiation on children, the health implications of long-term exposure to RF radiation, the ubiquity of wireless devices, and other technological developments that have occurred since the Commission last updated its guidelines, and

(iii) address the impacts of RF radiation on the environment."

The court did not impose a deadline for the FCC to respond to this mandate. As of this writing, the FCC has not yet responded to the court order.

Although the case is a procedural one, it has significant implications. It clarifies that FCC limits do not rest on an up to date science review and that federal agencies have dropped the ball. The public assumes that government scientists are researching and reviewing the latest science on cell phones, cell towers, Wi-Fi, 5G, and wireless networks to ensure safety limits remain adequate. Yet these assumptions are not based on reality. The reality is that federal agencies have not reviewed the totality of up to date research to ensure the public is protected.

No Scientific Review by Federal Agencies

The lack of federal agency activities regarding the health effects of RF is evidenced by the fact that not a single federal agency submitted a report or scientific review to the FCC record.

In its Inquiry, the FCC had directly written to several U.S. agencies with health and environmental expertise, asking them to submit comments with their opinions regarding RF limits.

Only the FDA responded with an opinion. The FDA simply submitted a short letter with one paragraph without substantiation, concluding that FCC limits were adequate.

Yet two months after the FCC made its decision to affirm the 1996 limits, the FDA then released an anonymous selective review of literature on brain cancer and wireless radiation. The issuance of an anonymous report by any federal agency with no reviewers is itself highly unusual. The FDA rejected entirely the National Toxicology Program animal study on cell phone radiation--the very study the FDA had requested in 1999 in order to gain information on human health impacts from long term exposure. The NTP study had found clear evidence of cancer as well as DNA damage.

The FDA had requested the NTP study in 1999 and reviewed it repeatedly throughout its conduct. The issuance of an anonymous report by any federal agency with no reviewers is highly unusual. However, ruling on procedural grounds, the court allowed the rejection of the cancer association but not all other health effects.

Furthermore, the court found the FCC's reliance on the FDA's "cursory" statements to be "unreasoned" because the FDA did not substantiate its opinion. The court found the FCC had improperly relied on conclusory statements and concluded that the FCC should have determined "how and why it (the FDA) reached its conclusions" as the FCC had a responsibility "to regulate radio communications

and devices that emit RF radiation and interfere with radio communications and to do so in the public interest, including in regard to
public health."

Other U.S. agencies such as the Department of Labor, EPA and
National Cancer Institute and the National Institute of Environmental
Health Sciences submitted short letters absent any research review or
scientifically supported opinion. Some of the agencies did not respond
at all. The FCC presented this silence as support for its determination.
The court did not agree.

Regarding a host of other alleged health impacts, including
impairment of male fertility, brain development, and effects on children, the court ruled the failure of agencies to submit anything to the
record cannot be construed as concurrence:

*Silence does not indicate why the expert agencies determined,
in light of evidence suggesting to the contrary, that exposure to
RF radiation at levels below the Commission's current limits does
not cause negative health effects unrelated to cancer. Silence does
not even indicate whether the expert agencies made any such
determination, or whether they considered any of the evidence in
the record.*

Wildlife Impacts Ignored

Among the many studies on pollinators that the FCC ignored was
a three-dimensional, anatomically-based model of the honeybee published in the distinguished journal, *Scientific Reports* by a team of European researchers. They found that the higher frequencies employed in
5G networks could uniquely resonate with the bodies of pollinating
insects, leading to significant increases in their exposure compared to
lower frequencies (Thielens et al. (2018)). The authors warned that this
resonance effect could overheat the insects bodies potentially leading to

major changes in insect behavior and physiology.

This team of honeybee researchers later published research on the absorption of 5G frequencies into honeybee models at various developmental and life stages: two worker bees, a drone, a larva, and the queen. They also took real-world measures of wireless radiation near beehives in Belgium and found that the expected shift in 5G to frequencies higher than 3 GHz would lead to an increase of honeybee absorption between 390–570 percent.

The survival of the entire hive depends on the vitality of its single queen that must be kept fed and healthy. Studies have also found that wireless radiation can impair the queen's capacity to lay eggs, produce broods, and survive winter torpor, putting entire hives at risk. Modern agriculture depends on more than 2,000 pollinating insects that already are in diminishing supply so that truckbeds of hives are sometimes driven into key ecological zones. While many factors underlie the declines of honeybees and other pollinators, including climate change, pesticides, and parasites, scientists are now warning that wireless radiation is also a significant factor.

Several scientific reviews have been published on a wide-range of wildlife impacts. A three-part landmark research review by B. Blake Levitt, former New York Times science reporter, Henry Lai, PhD, University of Washington professor emeritus and former Electromagnetic Biology and Medicine editor-in-chief, and Albert Manville, former senior scientist with the U.S. Fish and Wildlife Service, evaluated 1,200 peer-reviewed studies on the impacts of non-ionizing electromagnetic fields on flora and fauna concluding that, "broad wildlife effects have been seen on orientation and migration, food finding, reproduction, mating, nest and den building, territorial maintenance and defense, and longevity and survivorship."

The lack of consideration of wildlife and the natural environment is a critical regulatory gap. RF exposure limits are design for humans, not wildlife and trees. Birds nest on cell towers. 5G installations are being built right next to trees. No data are regularly gathered by environmental agencies to measure impacts to flora and fauna. No federal agency is reviewing the research on environmental impacts. Thus, the U.S. is still racing toward 5G without any consideration of the mounting science linking wireless radiation with a host of human, environmental and wildlife impacts.

Since 2019, several thousand more pages of scientific studies have been issued on the impacts of wireless radiation on wildlife and public health. It has been two years since the U.S. Circuit Court of Appeals for the District of Columbia ordered the agency to review the submitted record. Yet the FCC has remained silent.

U.S. Medical and Public Health Recommendations

Numerous medical and public health groups have issued recommendations to reduce exposure. In 2018, the American Academy of Pediatrics issued ten cell phone safety tips for families after the NTP animal study was released finding "clear evidence" that cell phone radiation increased two types of cancers in male rats and damaged DNA.

In 2017, after legal action by Dr. Joel Moskowitz, the California Department of Public Health (CDPH) released an advisory on reducing cell phone radiation. Public information requests revealed 27 drafts of the document going back to 2008 when the Environmental Health Investigations Branch of the California Department of Public Health began researching the issue. The 2009 draft of the California advisory included guidelines drafted by Drs. Ronald Herberman, EHT's first board chair, and Devra Davis, then-professor of epidemiology at the University of Pittsburgh School of Public Health and director of the University of Pittsburgh Cancer Institute's Center of Environmental Oncology.

Their report in 2007 included a section titled "What State Governments and Its Employees Can Do To Lower Potential Risks From Cordless Phones and Cell Phones." They also made timely recommendations to the primary purchasing arm of the federal government — the General Services Administration — on purchasing low-radiation equipment as well as recommendations on how employees can reduce exposure from cellular and cordless phones. State officials had been subject to industry pressures not to release the report. The document finally released had been radically loosened. Early and final versions of this advisory can be found on EHT's website.

That same year, the Maryland State Children's Environmental Health And Protection Advisory Council released a Wi-Fi in Schools Report recommending why and how schools could limit children's exposure to wireless radiation. A few years later, they released *Guidelines on How to Reduce EMF Exposure*. Both were the first-ever actions by an expert body of the state, including representatives from the Department of Health and other state organizations, elected officials, children's health experts, and pediatricians.

In 2023, the Santa Clara County Medical Association adopted best practice recommendations for technology in schools in order to educate physicians, school officials and teachers of the complex health risks and potential health hazards of digital and wireless technology in schools. The group examined research on the broad impacts of digital technology including health and neurologic effects of exposure to wireless radiation, eye effects, mental health effects and impacts on academic performance.

The New Hampshire Commission on 5G

While various states have tackled the lack of federal regulatory accountability and oversight in multiple ways, New Hampshire lawmakers made strides far and above the rest by creating an expert Commission to investigate the safety of 5G. Following a yearlong investigation with testimony from numerous U.S. and international experts, the commission issued a thorough well referenced "Final Report on 5G's Health and Environmental Effects."

The report reviewed the science and policy issues in the U.S. It offered clear recommendations for actions that government and industry can immediately do to reduce public exposure, raise awareness, and increase transparency. These are their key recommendations:

Strengthening regulations and addressing regulatory gaps

- A resolution by the U.S. Congress requiring the FCC to commission an independent health study and review safety limits.
- RF-radiation safety limits written by federal agencies with ecological knowledge that will protect trees, plants, birds, insects, and pollinators.
- An environmental impact statement by the FCC, under the National Environmental Policy Act, on the effects on New Hampshire and the country from 5G and the expansion of RF wireless technologies.
- New measurement protocols to evaluate high data rate signal characteristics associated with biological effects and summative effects of multiple radiation sources.

Reducing public exposure

- Enactment of a 1,640-foot cell antenna setback for homes and schools
- Replacement of Wi-Fi in schools and libraries with hardwired connections.
- Setbacks for new wireless antennas from residences, businesses, and schools.
- Deployment of fiber optic cable connectivity with wired con-

nections inside homes.
- Cell phones and wireless devices equipped with updated software to stop them from radiating when positioned against the body.
- Establishment of RF radiation-free zones in commercial and public buildings.

Raising public awareness
- Public service announcements on radio, television, and print by state health agencies to educate the public on minimizing RF exposure.
- Warnings by the state of New Hampshire regarding exposures to newborns, children, and pregnant women.

Increasing transparency
- Warning signs in commercial and public buildings.
- Publicly posted maps with information on radio frequency radiation level measures.
- Labeling of 5G structures for radio frequency radiation at eye level and making them readable from nine feet away.
- Independent contractors to perform RFR signal strength measurements for cell sites.
- Professional licensing and education for home inspectors so they can include RF intensity measurements in inspection reports.

Additional Actions Representatives Can Take

Elected officials' hands are not tied. Even if passing legislation seems impossible, representatives can use the power of their office to raise awareness. Officials can send letters to the FCC requesting they ensure protective, biologically based safety limits for wireless radiation. Officials can encourage the FCC to engage federal agencies with health and environmental expertise to develop science-based safety limits. Officials can also operate incrementally to make small strides that will eventually add up.

Local and State Actions

- Develop a protective wireless ordinance to restrict cell antennas near homes, schools, and workplaces.
- Ensure the location of all cell towers, small cells, and wireless facilities, along with the technical details and RF reports of current and proposed sites, are publicly posted so people are fully informed.
- Pass a resolution on cell phone and wireless radiation, informing the community about the issue and what they can do.
- Hold educational events in the community and distribute factsheets that raise awareness on steps families can take to reduce wireless exposure.
- Pass a resolution on electromagnetic sensitivity.
- Develop a list of recommended actions that can be taken in public spaces (libraries, schools, etc.) to accommodate people with electromagnetic sensitivity.
- Pass legislation that ensures consumers are aware of the measured RF radiation levels of cell phones and wireless devices and that cell phones and wireless devices emit radiation.
- Prioritize access to wired broadband to and through homes and workplaces.

Federal Actions

- A comprehensive national research program by the EPA on biological effects leading to the development of science-based exposure limits to protect the public, flora, and fauna.
- RF limits should be regularly reviewed by the EPA with up to date scientific evaluation.
- RF measurement and compliance protocols that consider the

complex signal characteristics associated with bio-effects and the cumulative effects from numerous sources.

- Evaluation of alternatives to SAR as the basis for limits. SAR is a heat-based metric and does not capture signal exposure characteristics relative to biological effects.
- Revisions to testing protocol for RF compliance of cell phones and wireless devices so that testing includes body-contact positions. Currently, devices are tested at various distances away *from the body*. Manufacturers can choose these distances, ranging from under one inch for cell phones to 8 inches for Wi-Fi routers, gaming consoles, and baby monitor bases. All wireless devices should be tested in real-world use patterns with child and pregnancy models.
- Launch a nationwide RF monitoring system. Electromagnetic field levels in the country must be measured and monitored over time, with all measurements posted and easily accessed by the public.
- An online map and registry for all cell towers, small cells, and wireless antenna base station installations.
- The FCC should develop a robust oversight and enforcement program with routine spot checks for RF compliance of cell towers and wireless facilities.
- All cell phones and wireless devices on the market should be periodically measured for RF compliance independent of company premarket compliance tests. Data should be posted on a public website where consumers can type in the make and model of their phones to get the RF measurements.
- Testing of new technologies and frequency bands for human safety and environmental effects before market deployment.
- Implement risk mitigation policies to reduce children's RF exposure: Until wireless radiation limits are scientifically

updated, measures must be in place to reduce exposure, especially for vulnerable populations. Measures could include a ban
on selling and advertising cell phones and wireless devices for
children, prohibition of cell towers on or near school properties,
and support for ethernet connections in schools and libraries.

- Requirements for RF levels and warning labels on mobile
  devices at the point of sale for cell phone and wireless device
  RF levels.

- Multimedia public service announcements on decreasing RF
  exposure, targeted at parents and pregnant women.

- Start a post market surveillance and reporting system for
  health and environmental impacts.

- Premarket test new technologies and frequencies for biological impacts and long term impacts before deployment

- Repeal Section 704 of the Telecom Act to enable municipal-
  ities to make their own decisions on the effects of radio frequency radiation and electromagnetic fields without the threat
  of lawsuits by telecom companies.

IV. Actions Industry Can Take To Reduce Exposure: Safer Choices and Design

Safer technology is possible. Solutions exist.

Wired networks, which are safer, faster, and more secure, must
be prioritized. The promotion of wired internet connections, rather
than everything wireless, will significantly reduce overall wireless
exposures to consumers and decrease environmental levels of
radiation.

At the same time, numerous hardware and software changes are
available that can significantly reduce RF exposure.

The International Commission on the Biological Effects of Electromagnetic Fields (ICBE-EMF) published an article in the *Interna-*

tional Journal of Environmental Research and Public Health that included several engineering fixes aimed at reducing users' cell phone radiation exposure, including:

1. Utilizing existing body sensors in Android and iPhone devices to automatically halt emissions when the phone is near the body.

2. Using antenna technologies with materials already patented by many cell phone manufacturers to reduce cell phone radiation exposure by 50-99 percent.

3. Eliminating cell phone "handshake" transmissions when the user and the user's phone are not moving.

4. Making airplane mode the default setting. Users can change the setting when they want to connect, but airplane mode automatically turns back on after a pause in use.

5. Developing applications to monitor and display cumulative call time, helping users limit the duration of their calls. One function could end calls (with appropriate warning) when a user's preset exposure limits are reached.

Other Actions Manufacturers Can Take To Minimize Cell Phone Radiation Exposure

- Provide several options for users to turn off all cell phone antennas at once, including an easy-to-find button, airplane mode, and powering off a device.

- Ensure that when powering on, all devices default to airplane mode with antennas off regardless of their status when the phone was turned off.

- Enable all cell phones and applications, including voice calls and text messages, as well as any other linked devices or accessories to be connected via wired lines (i.e., ethernet or other cables/cords).

- Provide ethernet adapters with all cell phones and other wireless-capable digital devices.
- Preset wireless antennas to shut off automatically when a device is connected via ethernet or other cabled or corded connections.
- Make manual updates the default position rather than having apps automatically and continually update.

What Manufacturers Can Do With Other Electronics

- Manufacture and market speakers and other audio-video gear, printers, and corded peripherals without wireless functionality.
- Equip products with wireless functionality to have a reliable physical switch to manually power off all wireless-emitting antennas.
- Make the default setting airplane mode with all antennas off.
- Make it possible for devices to easily plug into ethernet (so users don't always have to use Wi-Fi, Bluetooth, or other wireless connection methods).
- Set wireless antennas to be off automatically when corded connections are in use.
- Create an Eco-Function so that antennas turn off when not in use.
- Set all wireless antennas to go to the lowest power required to connect automatically rather than always be at the highest.
- Do not enable beacon signals to transmit constantly.

What Industry Can Do With Networks

- Deploy communications networks that run on robust wired networks to and though buildings instead of making everything wireless all the time.
- Support research and design focused on wired networks and corded equipment.
- Offer wired modems and wired routers inside the house that

match their systems "after the drop."

- Cable TV and internet providers should NOT be allowed to use customer routers as infrastructure that broadcasts network coverage outside the customer's premises to provide wireless service to other passersby unless the provider, in advance, specifically requests and receives permission from the customer.

The Basics of Reducing EMF in Building Construction, Renovation, and Outdoor Spaces

- Networks in buildings should be wired with convenient ethernet ports throughout each room and common area so that devices can be plugged into ports to access the internet, intranet, and other ICT networks; and with easy access for maintenance, repair, replacement, expansion, renovations, upgrades, etc.
- Corded phones (without wireless) should be standard in buildings.
- In outdoor spaces, public access to plug-in ports for portable devices should be provided to connect with ICT networks; these outdoor ports should be powered so that portable devices do not need to be self-powered (i.e., similar to the provision and accessibility of "pay phone" equipment and services).
- Magnetic and radio frequency electromagnetic fields should be regularly measured and mitigated.

V. International Policies to Minimize Children's Cell Phone and Wi-Fi Exposure.

Detailed references can be found at ehtrust.org.

Cell Phone Policy	Countries and Cities Taking Action
Straightforward official government agency advice that the public and/or children "should" minimize cell phone RF exposure.	United Kingdom, Russia, Switzerland, Finland, Ireland, Germany, Belgium, Greece, Israel, Turkey, Singapore, France, Denmark, India, Australia, Austria, Cyprus, Canada, Italy, French Polynesia, Korea, Sri Lanka, Croatia, Krakow Poland, European Parliament Resolution 1815
Public awareness program or campaign dedicated to educating the public on how to minimize RF.	France, French Polynesia, Israel, Italy, Cyprus, Tunisia, Israel
Ban on mobile phone advertising to children.	France, Belgium, French Polynesia, Russia
Ban on sale of phones designed for children.	Belgium, France, French Polynesia
SAR labeling (on the device, packaging, point of sale).	France, Israel, India, Belgium, Russia, Korea
A government agency with a surveillance program for cell phones and tests cell phones for SAR compliance.	France and Canada. A consortium of France, Greece, Latvia, Luxembourg, the Netherlands, and Switzerland began development of program in 2023
Wi-Fi in Schools	
Recommendations to prefer wired instead of Wi-Fi in kindergartens and schools.	France, Israel, Germany, French Polynesia, Salzburg, Austria, Maryland State Children's
	Environmental Health And Protection Advisory Council

Wi-Fi is banned in daycares and kindergartens.	Environmental Health And Protection Advisory Council
Wi-Fi is off or minimized in elementary schools.	France, Israel, Cyprus, and various municipal school districts worldwide
Cell Towers and Base Station Antennas	
Public exposure limits are more stringent than ICNIRP/FCC limits and/or policy for protective measures in "sensitive areas" (i.e., schools, daycares, and hospitals). For example, cell towers are prohibited near schools and/or more stringent RF limits in sensitive areas.	Italy, India, Israel, Chile, Croatia, Ukraine, Kuwait, Greece, China, Russia, Canada, Switzerland, Brussels, Belgium, Bosnia Herzegovina, Grand Duchy of Luxembourg, Greece, Belarus, Georgia, Serbia, Slovenia, Montenegro, Croatia, Bulgaria, Turkey, India, Liechtenstein, Tajikistan, Kazakhstan, Uzbekistan, Kyrgyzstan, Kuwait, Republic of Moldova, Iraq
Government measurement and monitoring program for cell tower RF and environmental RF exposures.	France, Greece, Turkey, Romania, Serbia, India, Israel, French Polynesia, Croatia, Bulgaria, Tunisia, Malta, Brazil, Bahrain, Monaco, Bhutan, Senegal, United Kingdom, Australia, Spain, Austria, India, Israel, Gibraltar, Brussels Belgium, Switzerland, Norway, Lithuania.

In addition to the list below, EHT has 5G and small cell briefing materials that include examples of protective ordinances and science related to policy. Please see more at ehtrust.org.

VI. Resources
Legal and Policy Resources

Harvard University Center for Ethics investigative journalist Norm Alster published the book *Captured Agency: How the Federal Communications Commission is Dominated by the Industries It Presumably Regulates* to document how the wireless industry uses Big Tobacco tactics.

Alster, N. (2015). *Captured Agency: How the Federal Communications Commission Is Dominated by the Industries It Presumably Regulates*. Edmond J. Safra Center for Ethics Harvard University. https://ethics.harvard.edu/files/center-for-ethics/files/capturedagency_alster.pdf

A chapter on cell tower radiation in the *Legal Handbook for Massachusetts' Board of Health, 3rd Edition* states, "Schools, houses of worship and commercial property owners can be considerable. The fact that towers are ubiquitous must not be confused with the presumption that they do not present certain health risks." The handbook highlights the legal issues, conflicting studies, and lack of consensus on safety.

Massachusetts Association of Health Boards. (2021). *The Legal Handbook for Massachusetts Boards of Health (3rd ed.)*. Massachusetts Association of Health Boards. https://www.mahb.org/wp-content/uploads/2021/05/Legal-Handbook-3rd-Edition-2021.pdf

The University of Pittsburgh Law Review published Hala Mouzaffar's "The FCC Keeps Letting Me Be: Why Radiofrequency Radiation Standards Have Failed to Keep Up With Technology," about how the FCC and FDA have failed in their obligations to prescribe safe RF guidelines to protect public health and safety.

Mouzaffar, H. (2021). "The FCC Keeps Letting Me Be: Why Radiofrequency Radiation Standards Have Failed to Keep Up With Technology." University of Pittsburgh Law Review, 83(1), Article 1. https://doi.org/10.5195/lawreview.2021.826

Former FCC lawyer Erica Rosenberg, who served as Assistant Chief of the Competition and Infrastructure Policy Division, published "Environmental Procedures at the FCC: A Case Study in Corporate Capture," detailing how the FCC has failed to follow environmental laws.

Rosenberg, E. (2022). "Environmental Procedures at the FCC: A Case Study in Corporate Capture. Environment: Science and Policy for Sustainable Development," 64(5–6), 17–27. https://doi.org/10.10 80/00139157.2022.2131190

Textbooks to Know

Davis, D., Sears, M. E., Miller, A. B., & Bray, R. (2017). *Microwave/Radiofrequency Radiation and Human Health: Clinical Management in the Digital Age.* In A. Cohen, F. S. vom Saal, & A. Weil (Eds.), Integrative Environmental Medicine (p. 0). Oxford University Press. https://doi.org/10.1093/med/9780190490911.003.0010

McDermott-Levy, R., Jackman-Murphy, K. P., Leffers, J., & Cantu, A. G. (Eds.). (2022). *Environmental Health in Nursing (2nd ed.).* Alliance of Nurses for Healthy Environments www.enviRN. org. https://envirn.org/wp-content/uploads/2022/05/Environmental-Health-in-Nursing-2nd-Ed-Final.pdf

Panagopoulos, D. J. (Ed.). (2022). *Electromagnetic Fields of Wireless Communications: Biological and Health Effects (1st ed.).* CRC Press. https://doi.org/10.1201/9781003201052

Davis, D., McCance, K. L., & Brashers, V. L. (2023). *Cancer Epidemiology. In McCance & Huether's Pathophysiology: The Biologic Basis for Disease in Adults and Children (9th ed., pp. 388–429).* Elsevier Health Sciences.

Markov, M. (2018). *Mobile communications and public health.* CRC Press.

Markov, M. S. (2015). *Electromagnetic fields in biology and medicine.* CRC Press.

Organizations and Websites

International Commission on the Biological Effects of Electromagnetic Fields (ICBE-EMF), icbe-emf.org

Physicians For Safe Technology, mdsafetech.org

Oceania Radiofrequency Science Advisory Association, orsaa.org

Canadians for Safe Technology, c4st.org

BioInitiative, bioinitiative.org

Americans for Responsible Technology, americansforresponsibletech.org

Grassroots Environmental Education, grassrootsinfo.org

BabySafe Project, babysafeproject.org

Prevent Cancer Now, preventcancernow.ca

PowerWatch, powerwatch.org.uk

Physicians' Health Initiative for Radiation and Environment, phiremedical.org

Manhattan Neighbors for Safer Telecommunication, manhattanneighbors.org

The Institute for Building-Biology® & Ecology, buildingbiologyinstitute.org

More organizations can be found at ehtrust.org

wildlifeandwireless.org

healthytechhome.org

Learn More
Joel M. Moskowitz, PhD, Director, Center for Family and Community Health, U.C. Berkeley School of Public Health has a blog, "Electromagnetic Radiation Safety," with science and policy on wireless and health at saferemr.com.

The Santa Clara County Medical Association (SCCMA) has published several articles about wireless impacts to wildlife, learning, and public health in its monthly bulletins written by Dr. Cindy Russell, a past president of the SCCMA. Dr. Russell was a longtime chair of its environmental health committee and founder of Physicians for Safe Technology.

Cell Phone Tower Locations in the U.S.
Go to Antenna Search at antennasearch.com and enter your address to find registered cell phone base station antennas. However, "small cells" and rooftop antennas are generally not listed on this site so check with your municipality.

VII. Research Studies To Know
Hundreds of studies indicating harmful effects have been published since *Disconnect* was published. In 2023, several distinguished experts in medicine, epidemiology, toxicology, physics, biochemical engineering, and public health and I coauthored a state-of-the-science review paper "Wireless Technologies, Non-ionizing Electromagnetic Fields and Children: Identifying and Reducing Health Risks." Collectively, we have published more than 2,000 papers. In this paper, we document the latest scientific research and recommend prudent approaches to reduce microwave radiation exposures to As Low As Reasonably Achievable (ALARA).

Here are a few of the essential research studies published over the last decade:

In 2011, radio frequency radiation was classified as a Class 2B possible carcinogen by the World Health Organization's International Agency for Research on Cancer. This classification applies to RF regardless of the source. Today, several scientists believe that the weight of current peer-reviewed evidence supports the upgraded conclusion that radio frequency radiation should now be regarded as a human carcinogen. See *Cancer Epidemiology Update*, Following The 2011 IARC Evaluation Of Radiofrequency Electromagnetic Fields (Monograph 102) published by Miller et al. (2018) and *Evaluation of Mobile Phone and Cordless Phone Use and Glioma Risk Using the Bradford Hill Viewpoints from 1965 on Association or Causation* by Hardell and Carlberg (2017).

In 2018, the U.S. National Toxicology Program (NTP) issued a final report on its $30 million animal studies finding that long-term cell phone radio frequency radiation exposure (two years) was associated with "clear evidence" of two types of cancers in male rats: glioma of the brain and schwannomas of the heart. These are the same types of cancer found in studies of people who heavily use cell phones up their heads. They also found RF exposure associated with reduced pup birth weights and the induction of cardiomyopathy of the right ventricle in male and female rats. Furthermore, the NTP's genotoxicity studies found "significant increases in DNA damage" in groups of mice and rats after just 14 to 19 weeks of exposure.

In 2018, the Ramazzini Institute published its findings from its large-scale animal study that used much lower exposure levels to mimic cell tower emission environmental levels. The exposed rats developed the same types of cancers as the U.S. National Toxicology Program found.

The European Parliament requested a research report. "Health Impact of 5G," released in July 2021, concluded that commonly used RF frequencies (450 to 6000 MHz) are probably carcinogenic for humans and affect male fertility with possible adverse effects on the development of embryos, fetuses, and newborns.

The Environmental Working Group published a study in *Environmental Health* titled "Development Of Health-Based Exposure Limits For Radiofrequency Radiation From Wireless Devices Using A Benchmark Dose Approach," analyzing the findings of tumor and heart damage from the U.S. National Toxicology Program study. It concluded that FCC limits should be strengthened 200 to 400 times to protect children.

Yale researchers published a study supported by the American Cancer Society linking thyroid cancer to cell phone use in people with a common genetic variation.

The Switzerland Institute of the Environment published "Manmade Electromagnetic Fields and Oxidative Stress — Biological Effects and Consequences for Health," a research review finding increased oxidative stress in the majority of animal studies and cell studies, even from exposures within regulatory limits.

A 2018 study simulating RF radiation exposure from virtual reality found that a child's eyes and brain regions can absorb 2 to 5 times higher levels than an adult's. "Absorption Of Wireless Radiation In The Child Versus Adult Brain And Eye From A Cell Phone Conversation Or Virtual Reality" by C. Fernández et al. was published in the journal *Environmental Research* in 2018.

"A Prospective Cohort Study of Adolescents' Memory Performance and Individual Brain Dose of Microwave Radiation from

Wireless Communication," a study on Swiss teenagers published in *Environmental Health Perspectives* by M. Foerster et al. (2018) found decreased memory among teenagers with higher cell phone exposures to the brain after one year, replicating an earlier study on teenagers.

"Evidence For A Health Risk by RF On Humans Living Around Mobile Phone Base Stations: From Radiofrequency Sickness To Cancer," a scientific literature review on cell tower base station antennas and human health, published in *Environmental Research* by Alfonzo Balmori documented that most studies found associations with radio frequency sickness, cancer, and changes in biochemical parameters.

A review paper titled "Limiting Liability With Positioning to Minimize Negative Health Effects of Cellular Phone Towers" by J.M. Pearce in 2020 reviewed the "large and growing body of evidence that human exposure to RFR from cellular phone base stations causes negative health effects." The authors recommend restricting antennas near homes and within 500 meters of schools and hospitals to protect companies from future liability.

A landmark three-part 2021 research review on effects on wildlife called "Effects of Non-ionizing Electromagnetic Fields on Flora and Fauna," published in *Reviews on Environmental Health* by U.S. experts, including former U.S. Fish and Wildlife senior biologist Albert Manville, states current science should trigger urgent regulatory action. It cited more than 1,200 scientific references that found adverse biological effects on wildlife from even very low intensities of non-ionizing radiation, with findings of impacts to orientation, migration, reproduction, mating, nest, den-building, and survivorship.

Sources of Information for the First Edition

Detailed linked references can be found online at ehtrust.org

Basic Background Resources

Robert Buderi, *The Invention That Changed the World: How a Small Group of Radar Pioneers Won the Second World War and Launched a Technological Revolution* (New York: Simon & Schuster, 1996), details the remarkable story of radar from its invention by British engineers as one of the major technological advances of the century, to its adaptation for mass production in MIT's famed rad lab (for radiation laboratory) in 1940. Aided by a massive investment in the United States and Britain, putting radar onto planes kept Britain from losing the war to Germany and provided an essential boost to the Allied war effort when the United States formally engaged.

Paul Brodeur, *The Zapping of America: Microwaves, Their Deadly Risk, and the Coverup* (New York: W. W. Norton, 1977), documented some of the hidden health risks of microwave radiation and efforts of the Defense Department and the electronics industry to keep these risks poorly understood.

Microwave News, a remarkable online documentation of major technical developments over the past thirty years, with interviews of many principal researchers, strongly expressed opinions about the principles and principals of the field, summaries of key findings, and unusually candid evaluations of personal, political, and scientific conflicts written, edited, and published by the irreverent investigative journalist Louis Slesin. www.microwave news.org

George Carlo and Martin Schram, *Cell Phones: Invisible Hazards in the Wireless Age* (New York: Avalon, 2001), offers the former head of the Wireless Technology Research effort's inside story of how he oversaw a six-yearlong, twenty-eight-million-dollar research program, with funds provided by the Cellular Telecommunications Industry Association, that did not yield important new information. After his research contract was not renewed, Carlo wrote this book, questioning the integrity of the cell phone industry and the government.

Devra Davis, *The Secret History of the War on Cancer*, paperback (New York: Basic Books, 2009), documents the social factors that influence the ability to conduct research on cell phones and the persistent spinning of inconvenient science.

Alan H. Frey, "From the Laboratory to the Courtroom: Science, Scientists, and the Regulatory Process," in Nicholas H. Steneck (editor), *Risk/Benefit Analysis: The Microwave Case* (San Francisco: San Francisco Press, 1982), pp. 197–228. Includes a candid exposé by one of the principal researchers in the field of the successful efforts to pull the plug on research on the Frey auditory effect and on studies of the blood-brain barrier.

Don Justesen, H. Ragan, L. Rogers, A. Guy, D. Hjeresen, W. Hinds, and R. Phillips, *Compilation and Assessment of Microwave Bioeffects: Final Report,* DOE Contract EY-76-C.06-1830, May 1978. This report recommended that government research be stopped on the blood-brain barrier, because conflicting results had been found — a recommendation that effectively shut off this critical line of research. In fact, the conflict over this research proved to be manufactured and distorted, as Frey indicated in his account of what went on behind the scenes to stifle independent inquiry in this field.

National Academy of Sciences, *Identification of Research Needs Relating to Potential Biological or Adverse Health Effects of Wireless*

Communication, chaired by Professor Frank Barnes, member of the National Academy of Engineering, 2008. This brief report noted the absence of a major national research program on cell phones and wireless technology, identified major data gaps and research priorities, and recommended a major program be carried out.

Thomas S. Kuhn, *The Structure of Scientific Revolutions* (Chicago and London: University of Chicago Press, 1996), provides the framework for understanding the normal work of routine science in contrast with the world-changing ideas of those who create new models of pursuing knowledge. Kuhn explains that scientific revolutionaries are not always heralded during their lifetimes and that scientists can be petty and argumentative about who gets credit for breakthroughs.

Derek J. de Solla Price, *Little Science, Big Science* (New York: Columbia University Press, 1963), contrasts the lone pursuit of new ideas by scientists of ancient times with the corporate approach taken increasingly by modern science.

Robert O. Becker and Gary Selden, *The Body Electric: Electromagnetism and the Foundation of Life* (New York: Harper, 1985), a well-written story of the author's painstaking discoveries of the existence of low levels of electric current in many biological media, ranging from a salamander's regrowing leg to a human brain cell in a Petri dish.

Robert O. Becker, *Cross Currents: The Perils of Electropollution, the Promise of Electromedicine* (New York: Jeremy P. Tarcher, Penguin, 1990, 2004), with preface by Louis Slesin, shows that electricity can benefit medicine by promoting bone healing, among other things, but also demonstrates that electricity can affect human health adversely.

Adam Burgess, *Cellular Phones, Public Fears, and a Culture of Precaution* (Cambridge: Cambridge University Press, 2004), a sociological analysis of the issues associated with cell phone concerns in different media in different nations for the past twenty years, highlighting institutional and cultural presumptions associated with these concerns.

B. Blake Levitt, *Electromagnetic Fields: A Consumer's Guide to the Issues and How to Protect Ourselves* (Orlando, Fl.: Harcourt Brace, 1995). A thorough overview of what is known and suspected about electromagnetic radiation including radio frequency radiation by this former award-winning New York Times science writer. The 2007 iUniverse Back in Print edition contains a new foreword by the author on the increasing ambient exposures from wireless technologies and their impacts on public health and the environment.

Lloyd Morgan and others, *Cellphones and Brain Tumors* —15 Reasons for Concern, can be found at ehtrust.org.

Kerry Crofton, *Wireless Radiation Rescue: Safeguard Your Family from Electropollution*, revised ed. (Toronto: Global Well Being Book, 2011), a self-published, broad overview of documented and suspected risks of cell phones, with concrete advice about risk reduction.

Technical Information and Studies on Cell Phones

At this point, the best overall source for such information is a German government-maintained site, www.emfportal.org. This site reveals that there are about six hundred total peer-reviewed studies using mobile phone-like exposures that are similar to those from today's pulsed, digital, smart phones or studying cell phones under real-life conditions.

Technical information on radio frequency radiation can be found on competing Web sites with different points of view, reflecting the priorities of sponsoring agencies and nonprofit groups ranging from activists to military and industrial groups and independent advisory groups that in fact are dependent on steady support and cooperation from those they seek to study.

General assurances that radio frequency radiation is unlikely to be harmful and that few precautionary policies are needed can be found on some government and major nonprofit-organization Web sites, such as this one from the European Commission's Scientific Committee on Emerging and Newly Identified Health Risks. Summary and full text of "Possible Effects of Electromagnetic Fields (EMF) on Human Health," the 2007 scientific assessment of the European Commission's SCENIHR WHO International EMF Program; and International Commission on Non-Ionizing Radiation Protection (ICNIRP).

In contrast, other official government pronouncements and nonprofit assessments advocate precautionary approaches, as does the European Environment Agency, headquartered in Copenhagen, which concludes that sufficient evidence exists of potential harm and that prudent avoidance should be adopted, as found in their official report on the subject: www.eea.europa.eu/highlights/radiation-risk-from. everyday-devices-assessed.

A comprehensive assessment of the field that promotes the precautionary approach was produced by David Carpenter, M.D., and Cindy Sage, a consultant in electromagnetic fields. The assessment, which is periodically updated, is published online at The BioInitiative Report, https://bioinitiative.org.

This view contrasts with that of the World Health Organization International EMF project, which was established in 1996 (https://who.int/initiatives/the-international-emf-project), has been extensively supported by industry and government funds, and is designed to review potential health effects and public concerns about growing exposure to this essential technology.

Industry maintains a database of studies and summaries of key developments that are available for private subscription of fifteen thousand dollars a year through either ELF Gateway or RF Gateway; this is overseen by the Electrical Power Research Institute, an independent, nonprofit company performing research, development, and demonstration in the electricity sector for the benefit of the public to which 90 percent of electrical utilities belong. This nonprofit company holds scientific meetings and sells exclusive information on radio frequency radiation that can only be used by its members.

In Britain, in 2002, Sir William Stewart, a distinguished physician, headed a national commission of public health experts that advised precautions should be taken about safe use of cell phones and that research should be carried out on children and adults. In 2010, the United Kingdom announced the long-term COSMOS project, which aims to study cell phone habits and health issues that may arise among 2.4 million cell phone users whose health will be followed over the next two decades.

Acknowledgments

The fact that this book arose is a credit, as is much of my life, to my parents, Jean and Harry B. Davis, who taught me to fight for what I believe in, and to my teachers in the Donora and Pittsburgh public schools and at the universities of Pittsburgh, Chicago, and Johns Hopkins, who gave me the tools to carry out this work.

My husband, Richard, remains the anchor of my life. People in industry and government offices worldwide have generously helped me carry out the research in this book; some of them must remain anonymous. They are heroes for reaching out to me and providing detailed information on the history and current workings of telecommunications devices today. I am fortunate to have a family, good colleagues, and dear friends who provide me with invaluable support to do the right thing at a time and on a topic for which such support is in short supply. I would never have written this analysis without critical encouragement provided by the University of Pittsburgh and the Heinz Endowments.

In addition to the inspiration of their lives, a few devoted critics have reviewed repeated drafts of this work and given sage counsel and unflinchingly candid advice: Lloyd Morgan, Ellie Marks, Harry Lehman, Wilhelm Mosgoeller, Ioannis Pandathis, and Elizabeth Kelley. Stephen Morrow, the executive editor at Dutton, believed in this work from the start and shaped it into — I hope — the kind of book my sister Sara Davis Buss said it had to be.

My agent, Al Zuckerman, of Writers House, kept me focused on the storyline within the grand picture. Production editor Julia Gilroy ensured accuracy and completeness.

Lorenzo Tomatis, the erudite former head of the International Agency for Research on Cancer (IARC) of the World Health Organization and a founder of the International Society of Doctors for the Environment, regularly encouraged my efforts and directed me to troves of documents in several languages regarding research on cell phones before his death in 2007.

For providing much sustenance and a wide variety of invaluable assistance, I also want to thank: Marcia Male, Frances Pollack, Yiping Hu, David Walls-Kaufman, Maryann Donovan, Kate Halsey, Franc Namba Kueda, Julia Heemstra, Jessica Nan, Casey McClellan, Susan Eriksen-Meier, Mikail Kogan, my son and daughter-in-law, Aaron and Donielle Morgenstern, and my daughter and son-in-law, Lea Morgenstern Baylis and Whitson Whiting Baylis.

Any errors this book contains are solely my responsibility. That there are not more of them is the result of the generous efforts of many patient colleagues, including Henry Lai, Alvaro de Salles, Om P. Gandhi, Franz Adlkofer, Frank Barnes, Dariusz Leszczynski, Ronald B. Herberman, Brian McKenna, David Servan-Schreiber, Annie Sasco, Katherine Henderson, Janette Sherman, Moe Mellion, Melissa Bondy, Cindy Sage, Peggy Bare, Hattie and Leon Bradlow, Bill Bruno, Stan Hartman, Camilla Rees, and Vic Edgerton. Also, the scientists from the International EMF Scientist Appeal provide a stalwart resource for me and many others.

I have learned much from my colleagues at a number of institutions, some of which have provided direct support for my research, including the American Association for the Advancement of Science, the American Holistic Medical Association, the American Medical Women's Association, University of California, Baylor College of Medicine, the American Public Health Association, the New York

Academy of Sciences, Breast Cancer Fund, the Coalition of Organizations on the Environment and Jewish Life, Jackson Haverim, Beth Shalom Library Minyan, Adas Israel Synagogue's Havera, the Canadian Cancer Society, Cancer Care Ontario, the Children's Health and Environment Coalition, the Coalition of Organizations on the Environment and Jewish Life, Collegium Ramazzini, the Conservative Women's League, Hadassah, Harvard University, Johns Hopkins University School of Public Health, the London School of Hygiene and Tropical Medicine, the Pan American Health Organization, the Pittsburgh Jewish Community Center, the United Jewish Federation of Pittsburgh Environmental Committee, the Jackson Hole Jewish Community, and the Capitol Hill Havera. Thank you to Eleanor H. whose identity has been changed to protect her.

Thanks to the librarians who have helped me, in particular, Carol Conners and her colleagues at the Teton County Library, the archives and film collection of the National Library of Medicine, the Medical and Historical Collections of the University of Pittsburgh Medical and College Libraries, the Morgantown Public Library, West Virginia, Library of the National Institute of Occupational Safety and Health, and the generous, spirited archivists and reference experts of the Carnegie Library of Pittsburgh, one of the nation's oldest public libraries and one of the few that fortunately remains open some part of the weekend.

I doubt that it would have been possible to complete this work without the good graces of the Library of Congress Photographic Services Department or access to the archives of the American Association for the Advancement of Science. Those who set up and maintain EPA's websites, and who staffed and operated its now-closed libraries, deserve medals, as do scores of its dedicated, under-recognized employees, and those of the Centers for Disease Control and Prevention, the Occupational Safety and Health Administration, the

Food and Drug Administration, and the Federal Communications Commission.

The Environmental Health Trust (EHT) is my cherished vehicle for putting ongoing scientific work and discoveries into the public domain. It truly takes a village. My heartfelt thanks to the entire EHT family: our tireless Executive Director, Theodora Scarato, who constitutes a walking encyclopedia of ongoing efforts to promote safer technology and has developed the simple steps needed to protect our families featured in the final section of this new edition, our Chief Operating Officer, Sharon Kehnemui, who is wrenching order from our creative chaos, the mega-talented Debbie ONeal, and the astonishingly resourceful and ever-patient Candace Woodbury. Paul Ben-Ishai consistently provides cogent explanations of complex phenomena, despite a demanding academic schedule. Barbara Payne has offered invaluable eagle-eyed editing to these and many other pages. Judy Katz remains one of a kind — a valued, trusted, and savvy advisor whose wisdom infuses our efforts. A longtime friend, enthusiastic fellow-writer, and creative publicist, Judy unstintingly turns many a rainy day bright.

EHT is fortunate to have the wisdom of our distinguished board of directors, led by Chairman Hugh Taylor MD, chief of obstetrics and gynecology at Yale Medical Center; Secretary/Treasurer and global energy guru Tom Factor; Hillel Baldwin MD, AANS, recently retired after four decades in neurosurgery; Aly Cohen MD, tripled boarded in immunology, internal, and integrative medicine, and author of *Dr. Weil's Healthy Living Guide, Non-Toxic Guide to Living Healthy in a Chemical World*; Lendri Purcell, the visionary vice president of Jonas Philanthropies and Founder of Families Advocating for Chemical and Toxics Safety; and Angela Zener, social business and strategic digital media advisor. For a decade, Morris Mellion MD, skillfully served as chair and is now chairman emeritus of EHT. He and his intrepid wife Irene provided detailed criticism of the first edition of *Discon-*

nect. Along with Roxanne and Tom Factor, they dispensed invaluable guidance and considerable nourishment. Linda Birnbaum, former director of the National Institute of Environmental Health Sciences and a lifelong friend and colleague, remains a dear trusted advisor, along with my longtime collaborator, the prolific Anthony B. Miller, my newly found old friends, David Gee, Kent Chamberlin, Ron Melnick, and many other members of the International Commission on the Biological Effects of Electromagnetic Fields.

Lucy R. Wiletzky believed in this project years ago and has consistently supported our efforts intellectually and financially. George Klabin has provided important contributions to various EHT efforts to promote better public understanding of why and how to reduce wireless radiation, goading us to reach farther. Attorney Edward B. Myers, now retired, in his determination to have the courts compel the FCC to read the science, proved you can always stand on the truth, as have. attorneys, Robert Berg, Julian Gresser, Hunter Lundy, Erica Rosenberg, Joseph Sandri, and Dana. Grants from the Klungness Foundation, the Carroll Petrie Foundation, Jonas Philanthropies, Dr. Myron and Prudence Wentz, Ruth Westreich Foundation, the Klungness Foundation, and several generous anonymous donors and thousands of other private donors sustain our efforts. For more than a decade the Community Foundation of Jackson Hole has consistently and generously supported our efforts to provide local multimedia information that has become the model for communities around the world.

This new edition is occasioned by the remarkable growth of science confirming the need to reduce exposures to wireless radiation. This second edition is dedicated to three important groups.

My five rambunctious, talented, and ebullient grandchildren, Davis, Josephine, Raleigh, Noa Jane, and Ruby, with fervent hopes that they and their progeny will live in a safer and healthier world because of the efforts begun here.

Then to the mounting roster of those who are no longer with us, never imagining that the way they used cell phones or other wireless devices might shorten their lives, with the hope that through this book there will be fewer of them in the future.

Finally, to the growing numbers of brave and bold scientists around the world who are speaking out regarding the harms that can be prevented and to the wonderful community warriors in North America and from Brazil to Belgium, from Australia to Amsterdam, from India to Israel, from Paris to Panama, from New York to Nairobi who are translating that science into practical advice.

Last but far from least, to the Holy One who has allowed me to reach this season, I give whatever thanks can be rendered by mere words alone. To my grandchildren, I offer the hopes and dreams of grandparents everywhere — may you be blessed with undamaged brains, bodies, and souls, in part because of the work that this book continues.

ABOUT THE AUTHOR

D avis has held a number of academic posts, including, Gottes-
man Distinguished Visiting Professor, Yeshiva University;
Honorary Professor, London School of Hygiene and Trop-
ical Medicine; Visiting Professor of Medicine, Hadassah Medical
School, Mt. Sinai School of Medicine NYC; Ondokuz Mayis Medical
School, Samsun, Turkey; and Visiting Professor, Sichuan University,
Chengdu, China.

A National Book Award finalist for When Smoke Ran Like Water,
Devra Davis, Ph.D., MPH, is also the critically acclaimed author of The
Secret History of the War on Cancer, and Founder and President of the
Environmental Health Trust (EHT), a scientific and policy think tank.

Published in a dozen languages, *Disconnect* was awarded the
Nautilus Silver Medal for courageous investigation in 2013. Davis is
the founding executive director of both the Board on Environmental
Studies and Toxicology of the National Academy of Sciences and the
Center for Environmental Oncology of the University of Pittsburgh

Cancer Institute, where she was also Professor of Epidemiology. Scientific journal editor and author of more than 220 scientific publications and numerous blogs, Davis is a member of the team awarded the Nobel Peace Prize with Al Gore in 2007 and winner of the Green America Lifetime Achievement award for distinguished contributions to Public Health and the Carnegie Science Medal. Her TEDx talk and Melbourne University lectures have reached more than 11 million views.

A leader of President Clinton's National Action Plan on Breast Cancer, she lectures at numerous universities and academies of sciences and medicine around the world as well as at Harvard, Yale, the University of California, and other global institutions and has advised the Centers for Disease Control and Prevention, World Health Organization, World Bank, United Nations Development Program, and others. Featured on CNN, ABC, FOX, CBC, CCTV and major networks in Australia, India, England, and Europe, she and her husband live in Jackson Hole, Wyoming, and Washington, DC.

Davis received her B.S. and M.A. in 1967 from the University of Pittsburgh. Awarded Danforth Graduate Teaching Fellowship for the University of Chicago, where she completed her doctoral studies and a National Cancer Institute Senior Post-doctoral fellowship for outstanding service by the Director of the National Cancer Institute, and numerous accolades for her fearless and often ground-breaking scientific writing on environmental health, she is also a member of Pittsburgh's Taylor Allderdice High School Hall of Fame

Awarded her B.S. and M.A. from the University of Pittsburgh in 1967, Davis completed her interdisciplinary doctoral studies as a Danforth Foundation fellow at the University of Chicago in 1972, and her post-doctoral MPH from Johns Hopkins University as a Senior National Cancer Institute Fellow.

A member of the American College of Eben neology fellow of the Collegium Ramazzini — an international Public Health honorary society.

Other Books by the Author

- Ng, Lorenz K. Y.; Davis, Devra Lee, eds. (1981). *Strategies For Public Health: Promoting Health and Preventing Disease.*
- Davis, Devra Lee; Hoel, David, eds. (1990). *Trends in Cancer Mortality in Industrial Countries.*
- Davis, Devra (2002). *When Smoke Ran Like Water: Tales of Environmental Deception and the Battle Against Pollution.*
- Davis, Devra (2007). *The Secret History of the War on Cancer.*

Index

The United Nations Environment Programme (UNEP) 254
University of Athens 87
University of Pittsburgh Cancer Institute 110
University of South Florida 178
University of Szeged 163
University of Utah 99–101, 109
University of Washington 218
U.S. Circuit Court of Appeals 286
U.S. Congress 70, 127, 230, 241
U.S. Department of Defense
  and Beischer's research 176
  and Boland's research 233–235
  and COMAR 136
  and Gandhi's research 101–103
  and the FDA 69–71
  and university-based research 132
  and weapons research 138
U.S. Department of Energy 137
U.S. Food and Drug Adminstration (FDA)
  and conflicting reports on studies 69
  and microwave oven testing 226–227
  and safety testing 69
  and the CTIA 194
  and warning labels 237
  industry influence on 190
  Slesin on 183
U.S. National Institute of Environmental Health Sciences 230
U.S. Navy, See also Office of Naval Research 57
U.S. Office of Research and Development 61

V

V-2 rockets 58
Verizon 233
Verne, Jules 43, 50
video recordings 30
visible light 46
vision problems 212–215
Vodafone Foundation 140
Volkov, Nora 260–264

W

Wallace, Alfred R. 78

Wall-E 40
Walter Reed Army Medical Center 133
Waters, Bob 180
Watson, Diane 110
Watson, James C. 79
weather radar 63
Wheeler, Tom 196
William Stewart 225
Wilson, Robert 49
wireless headsets 155, 235, 309
Wireless Technology Research Limited Liability Company (WTR) 127, 196–197, 207, 230, 243–244
World Health Organization (WHO)
  and Brundtland 36, 73–75
  and the CTIA 194
  and the Verum Foundation 127
  International Agency for Research on Cancer 211
  Interphone study 75, 202–206, 210–211, 216–218, 218, 231, 262
  on risk of electromagnetic exposure 98
World War I 58–59
World War II
  and atomic weapons 188
  and magnetron development 60–64
  and microwave research 64–67
  and radar 57–63
  and sonar 57
  and X-ray technology 35
  ophthalmology research 212

X

X-rays 35, 45, 45–47, 79

Y

young adults, See also children; teenagers 35, 160, 204, 217, 231

Z

The Zapping of America 80, 136
Zaret, Milton M. 212–213

Made in United States
Troutdale, OR
03/14/2024

18450175R00216